Second Edition

Board of Registry Study Guide

Practice Questions for the Histotechnology Examinations

Second Edition

Board of Registry Study Guide

Practice Questions for the Histotechnology Examinations

Editor:

Freida L. Carson, Ph.D., HT(ASCP)

Associate Editors:

Laura Culver Edgar, MBA, MT(ASCP)

Donna Surges Tatum, Ph.D.

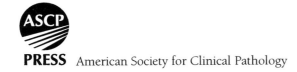

PRESS American Society for Clinical Pathology

Printed in the United States of America

07 06 05   7 6 5 4

Contents

Introduction

The Board of Registry (BOR) of the American Society of Clinical Pathologists and the National Society for Histotechnology (NSH) have worked together to prepare this 2nd edition for those preparing for the certification examination for histologic technicians and histotechnologists. This updated edition contains information on the Board of Registry; guidelines for preparing for and taking the test; information on the development, content, structure, and scoring of the examinations; and practice questions and answers in the content areas covered by the examinations.

The practice questions are presented in a format and style similar to the questions included in the Board of Registry certification examinations. These practice questions were compiled from previously published materials and individually submitted questions.

NONE OF THESE QUESTIONS WILL APPEAR ON ANY BOARD OF REGISTRY EXAMINATION.

Use of this book does not assure a passing score on the examinations. The Board of Registry's evaluation and credentialing process are entirely independent of this study guide. However, this book should help you prepare for the actual examination.

This book also provides information on how Board of Registry certification examinations are structured and scored. The technical summaries on these topics are designed to briefly explain the pertinent evaluation topics.

Reading List

This list is intended only as a partial reference source. Its distribution does not indicate endorsement by the Board of Registry of the American Society of Clinical Pathologists, nor does the Society wish to imply that the content of the examination will be drawn solely from these publications.

General Histotechnology

Allen K, for the American Society for Cytotechnology. *A Guide to Cytopreparation*. Chicago, IL: ASCT Press; 1998.

Bancroft JD, Horobin RW. *Troubleshooting Histology Stains*. New York, NY: Churchill-Livingstone, Inc.; 1998.

*Bancroft JD, Stevens A. *Theory and Practice of Histological Techniques*. 4th ed. New York, NY: Churchill-Livingstone, Inc.; 1996.

Burkitt HG, Young B, Heath JW. *Wheater's Functional Histology*. 3rd ed. New York, NY: Churchill-Livingstone, Inc.; 1993.

Carson F. *Histotechnology: A Self-Instructional Text*. 2nd ed. Chicago, IL: ASCP Press; 1997.

National Society of Histotechnology. *Journal of Histotechnology*. 4201 Northview Dr, Suite 502, Bowie, MD 20716-1073.

Sheehan D, Hrapchak B. *Theory and Practice of Histotechnology*. 2nd ed. Columbus, OH: Battelle Press; 1987.

Study Guide & Self-Assessment Booklets

Carson F. *Histotechnology: A Self-Assessment Workbook*. Chicago, IL: ASCP Press; 1997.

Histotechnology Examinations: Board of Registry Study Guide. Chicago, IL: ASCP Press; 2001.

Michigan Society of Histotechnologists. *HT/HTL Study Guide*, 1995 Edition—c/o Michelle Conrad, 269-668-2726.

National Society of Histotechnology. *Self-Assessment Examination Booklets*. 4201 Northview Dr., Suite 502, Bowie, MD 20716-2604.

Management

*Klosinski DD, Wallace MA. *Clinical Laboratory Science Education and Management*. Philadelphia, PA; W.B. Saunders; 1997.

*Varnadoe LA: *Medical Laboratory Management and Supervision, Operations, Review and Study Guide*. Philadelphia, PA: F.A. Davis Company; 1996.

Please refer to NSH: *Educational Resources in Histotechnology* for additional pertinent reading material.

---

*These references are more appropriate for the HTL level.

Chapter 1

Certification

The Importance of Certification

The practice of modern medicine would be impossible without the tests performed in the laboratory. A highly skilled medical team of pathologists, specialists, technologists, and technicians works together to determine the presence, extent, or absence of disease and provides valuable data needed to evaluate the effectiveness of treatment.

Today's laboratory uses many complex, precision instruments and a variety of automated and electronic equipment. However, the success of the laboratory begins with the laboratorians' dedication to their profession and willingness to help others. Laboratorians must produce accurate and reliable test results, have an interest in science, and be able to recognize their responsibility for affecting human lives.

Certification is the process by which a nongovernmental agency or association grants recognition of competency to an individual who has met certain predetermined qualifications, as specified by that agency or association. Certification affirms that an individual has demonstrated that he or she possesses the knowledge and skills to perform essential tasks in the medical laboratory. The Board of Registry certifies those individuals who meet academic and clinical prerequisites and who achieve acceptable performance levels on examinations.

Role of the ASCP Board of Registry

Founded in 1928 by the American Society of Clinical Pathologists (ASCP), the Board of Registry, as the preeminent certification agency in the field of laboratory medicine, promotes the health and safety of the public. Composed of representatives of professional organizations and the public, the Board's mission is to: 1) certify the competency of laboratory personnel, 2) set the standard for quality examination development and administration, 3) assist educational programs in evaluating their effectiveness, 4) perform research on and develop methods of competency evaluation, 5) provide study materials for examination preparation, and 6) maintain a registry of certified individuals.

The Board of Registry consists of more than 100 volunteer technologists and technicians, laboratory scientists, physicians, and professional researchers. These volunteers contribute their time and expertise to the Board of Governors, the Research and Development Committee, and the examination committees. These individuals help the BOR strive toward its goal of achieving excellence in the certification process for medical laboratory personnel.

The Board of Governors is the policy-making body for the Board of Registry and is composed of twenty-one members. These twenty-one members include technologists, technicians, and pathologists nominated by the ASCP and representatives from the general public and the following societies: the American Association for Clinical Chemistry, the American Association of Blood Banks, the American College of Microbiology, the American Society of Cytopathology, the American Society of Hematology, the Clinical Laboratory Management Association, and the National Society for Histotechnology.

The Board of Registry's Research and Development Committee's activities include the review of current methods and research related to competency definition, test development, validity and reliability assessment, examination performance, and standard setting. This committee is also actively involved in a 10-year prospective study of medical technologists.

The examination committees are composed of technicians, technologists, clinical scientists, and pathologists. These committees are responsible for the planning, development, and review of the examination databases; determining the accuracy and relevancy of the questions; and confirming the standard for each examination.

After Certification

Registration is the process by which names of individuals certified by the Board of Registry are identified on an annual basis as being currently registered. Annual registration benefits include an identification card, registration seal, one-year subscription to *Laboratory Medicine*, eligibility for insurance programs, and free copies of certification documents.

Certification in a given category means that an individual has met all criteria for career entry in that category. As they continue on in their careers, many individuals who are certified at one professional level may work to obtain certification at a higher level to reflect their continued growth and development. Thus, a technician may move to the technologist level and even to the specialist level in some disciplines.

Medical laboratory sciences are among the fastest-changing segments of the health care field. Therefore, each certificant should embrace a philosophy of lifelong learning to remain current in his or her chosen discipline. This may be accomplished through the Board of Registry's Continuing Competence Recognition Program, formal course work, professional continuing education offerings, and/or individual regimens of journal reading and subscription to professional self-assessment examinations.

Chapter 2

Technician and Technologist Certification

The Board of Registry's professional levels of practice were first compiled in 1982 (*Laboratory Medicine*, 1982;13:312-313). They were updated in 1993 and again in 1998 under the direction of the Board of Governors and the Research and Development Committee. These professional levels define in a general sense the skills and abilities that an individual is expected to have at career entry. Career entry is defined as that point in time when an individual meets all educational and/or supervisory requirements of the Board of Registry and is therefore eligible for Board Certification. The professional levels are considered hierarchical; that is, each level encompasses the knowledge and skill of the preceding level.

Technician Level

Knowledge
The technician has a working comprehension of the technical and procedural aspects of laboratory tests. The technician maintains awareness and complies with safety procedures and ethical standards of practice. The technician correlates laboratory tests to disease processes and understands basic physiology, recognizing appropriate test selection and abnormal test results.

Technical Skills
* *Follows established procedures for collecting and processing biological specimens for analysis.*

The technician comprehends and follows procedural guidelines to perform laboratory tests, including: (1) specimen collection and processing, (2) instrument operation and troubleshooting, (3) result reporting and record documentation, (4) quality control monitoring, (5) computer applications, and (6) safety requirements.

Problem Solving and Decision Making
* *Recognizes unexpected results and instrument malfunction and takes appropriate action.*

The technician recognizes the existence of procedural and technical problems and takes corrective action according to predetermined criteria or refers the problem to the appropriate supervisor. The technician prioritizes test requests to maintain standard patient care and maximal efficiency.

Communication
- *Provides laboratory information to authorized sources.*

The technician communicates specimen requirements, reference ranges, and test results, and prepares drafts of procedures for laboratory tests according to a standard format.

Teaching and Training Responsibilities
- *Demonstrates laboratory technical skills to other laboratory personnel.*

The technician trains new technicians and students and maintains technical competence.

Technologist Level

Knowledge
The technologist has an understanding of the underlying scientific principles of laboratory testing as well as the technical, procedural, and problem-solving aspects. The technologist has a general comprehension of the many factors that affect health and disease, and recognizes the importance of proper test selection, the numerous causes of discrepant test results (patient and laboratory), deviations of test results, and ethics including result confidentiality. The technologist correlates abnormal laboratory data with pathologic states determines validity of test results and need for additional tests. The technologist understands and enforces safety regulations, uses statistical methods, and applies business and economic data in decision-making. The technologist has an appreciation of the roles and an interrelationship of paramedical and other health-related fields, and follows the ethical code of conduct for the profession.

Technical Skills
- *Participates in the evaluation of new techniques and procedures in the laboratory.*

The technologist is capable of performing and interpreting standard, complex, and specialized tests. The technologist has an understanding of quality assurance sufficient to implement and monitor quality control programs. The technologist is able to participate in the introduction, investigation, and implementation of new procedures and in the evaluation of new instruments. The technologist evaluates computer-generated data and troubleshoots problems. The technologist understands and uses troubleshooting, validation, statistical, computer, and preventive maintenance techniques to insure proper laboratory operation.

Problem Solving and Analytical Decision Making
- *Evaluates and solves problems related to collection and processing of biological specimens for analysis.*
- *Differentiates and resolves technical, instrument, physiologic causes of problems or unexpected test results.*

The technologist has the ability to exercise initiative and independent judgment in dealing with the broad scope of procedural and technical problems. The technologist is able to participate in, and may be delegated, the responsibility for decisions involving: quality control/quality assurance programs, instrument and methodology selection, preventive maintenance, safety procedures, reagent purchases, test selection/utilization, research procedures, computer/statistical data.

Communication

- *Provides administrative and technical consulting services on laboratory testing.*

The technologist communicates technical information, such as answering inquiries regarding test results, methodology, test specificity and sensitivity, and specific factors that can influence test results to other health professionals and consumers. The technologist develops acceptable criteria, laboratory manuals, reports, guidelines, and research protocols.

Teaching and Training Responsibilities

- *Incorporates principles of educational methodology in the instruction of laboratory personnel, other health care professionals, and consumers.*

The technologist provides instruction in theory, technical skills, safety protocols, and application of laboratory test procedures. The technologist provides continuing education for laboratory personnel and maintains technical competence. The technologist may participate in the evaluation of the effectiveness of educational programs.

Supervision and Management

- *Gives direction and guidance to technical and support personnel.*

The technologist has an understanding of management theory, economic impact, and management functions. The technologist participates in and takes responsibility for establishing technical and administrative procedures, quality control, quality assurance, standards of practice, safety and waste management procedures, information management, and cost-effective measures. The technologist supervises laboratory personnel.

Chapter 3

Applying for the Certification Examination

The HT and HTL certification examinations have 2 parts: a multiple-choice examination and a practical component. Candidates must complete both components successfully to earn certification.

The 100-question multiple-choice examination is administered on computer. Computerized testing is offered in 4 examination cycles. These cycles are on a recurring quarterly basis: January-March; April-June; July-September; and October-December. The Board of Registry conducts 2 histology practical grading sessions per year—one in May and one in November.

Approximately one year before the date you wish to take the examination, you should contact the Board of Registry to obtain a current application packet. In addition to the application form, the application packet includes the *Procedures for Examination and Certification*. This booklet contains the application deadlines and examination dates, the examination eligibility requirements, and a list of test centers. Because the examination requirements, as well as other information included in the application packet, are periodically revised, be sure you have the most recent application packet available from the Board of Registry office. Once you have obtained these materials, it is important to review them to make sure that you have adequate time to obtain any required documents prior to the application deadline. Upon receipt of your application form, practical examination instructions will be mailed to you. Please contact the Board of Registry office at P.O. Box 12277, Chicago, Illinois 60612-0277, for application forms and general information. This information is also available on our web site at: www.ascp.org/bor.

Application Deadlines

Your application and fee for taking the computer adaptive test must be postmarked by January 1 (for the April-June exam cycle); April 1 (for the July-September exam cycle); July 1 (for the October-December exam cycle); and October 1 (for the January-March exam cycle for the following year).

For the practical component of the HT and HTL examinations, the application deadlines are: January 1 (for May OR November); April 1 (for November OR May of the following year); July 1 (for November OR May of the following year); and October 1 (for either May OR November of the following year).

Examination Eligibility

To be eligible to take the examination, you must 1) meet the current stated minimum requirements for a particular category or level of certification, and 2) submit a formal application form and pay the appropriate fee. The minimum requirements for each examination are summarized in TABLE 1. For detailed information, refer to the current Board of Registry Eligibility Requirements.

Table 1: Summary of the Eligibility Requirements for BOR Examinations

Certification	Requirements
Medical Technologist (MT)	Baccalaureate degree and one of the following: 1) NAACLS-accredited MT program OR 2) MLT(ASCP) certification and 3 years experience OR 3) 5 years experience
Medical Laboratory Technician (MLT)	Associate degree and one of the following: 1) NAACLS-accredited MLT program OR 2) CLA(ASCP) certification OR 3) completion of a 50-week military Medical Laboratory training course OR 4) 3 years experience
Histologic Technician (HT)	High school diploma and one of the following: 1) NAACLS-accredited HT program OR 2) Associate degree and 1 year experience OR 3) 2 years experience (As of 2005 route will be discontinued. The last application deadline for this route will be July 1, 2004.)
Histotechnologist (HTL)	Baccalaureate degree and one of the following: 1) NAACLS-accredited HT program OR 2) 1 year experience
Categorical Certification (BB,C,H,I,M)	Baccalaureate degree and one of the following: 1) MT (ASCP) certification OR 2) 2 years experience OR 3) Master's degree and 6 months experience
Cytotechnologist (CT)	Baccalaureate degree and CAAHEP-accredited CT program
Specialist in Cytotechnology (SCT)	CT(ASCP) certification and one of the following: 1) Baccalaureate degree and 5 years experience OR 2) Master's degree and 4 years experience OR 3) Doctorate degree and 3 years experience
Specialist in Blood Banking (SBB)	One of the following: 1) Baccalaureate degree and CAAHEP-accredited SBB program OR 2) Baccalaureate degree, MT(ASCP) or BB(ASCP) certification, and 5 years experience OR 3) Master's or Doctorate degree and 3 years experience
Specialist Certification (SBB,SC,SH,SI,SM)	One of the following: 1)Baccalaureate degree, Technologist certification, and 5 years experience OR 2) Master's degree and 4 years experience OR 3) Doctorate degree and 2 years experience
Specialist in Laboratory Safety (SLS)	One of the following: 1) Technologist or Specialist certification and 1 year experience OR 2) MLT(ASCP) or HT(ASCP) and 18 months experience OR 3) baccalaureate degree and 2 years experience
Specialist in Virology (SV)	One of the following: 1) SM(ASCP) certification and 1 year experience OR 2) MT(ASCP) or M(ASCP) certification and 2 years experience OR 3) Baccalaureate degree and 5 years experience OR 4) Master's degree and 4 years experience
Diplomate in Laboratory Management (DLM)	Baccalaureate degree, Master's degree, or Doctorate, and appropriate laboratory management education and experience
Phlebotomy Technician (PBT)	High school graduation (or equivalent) and one of the following: 1) completion of NAACLS-approved phlebotomy program OR 2) completion of acceptable phlebotomy program at a regionally accredited college/university or accredited laboratory OR 3) 1 year of full-time experience in an accredited laboratory OR 4) completion of other accredited allied health professional/occupational education
Hemapheresis Practitioner (HP)	One of the following: 1) RN and 3 years experience OR 2) MT(ASCP), BB(ASCP), OR SBB(ASCP) certification and 3 years experience OR 3) Baccalaureate degree and 5 years experience.

Chapter 4

Preparing to
Take the Examination

Begin early to prepare for the Certification Examination. Because of the broad range of knowledge and skills tested by the examination, even applicants with college training and professional experience will probably find that some review is necessary, although the amount will vary from applicant to applicant. Generally, last-minute cramming is the least effective method for preparing for the examination. The earlier that you begin, the more time you will have to prepare; and the more you prepare, the better your chance of doing well on the examination.

The following are some guidelines for studying for the examination.

Study for the Test

Plan a course of study that allows more time for your weaker areas. Although it is important to study in your areas of weakness, be sure to allow enough time to review all areas.

It is better to spend a short time studying every day than to spend several hours every week or two. Setting aside a regular time and a special place to study will help because studying will then become a part of your daily routine.

Several resources can be used to help you to study. The reading lists at the end of this book identify many useful books by subject area. The most current reading lists for the examinations are available on the ASCP's Web site at: www.ascp.org/bor. The practice questions in this book and provide an extensive overview of histotechnology questions. It can be used to test your knowledge in each subject area or to acquire experience in answering multiple-choice questions. You may also wish to consider using the following materials as study aids:

Standard Textbooks
Textbooks tend to cover a broad range of knowledge in a given field and thus help you survey an entire field. An added benefit is that textbooks frequently have questions at the end of the chapters that you can use to test yourself.

Competency Statements and Content Outlines
The Board of Registry has developed competency statements and content outlines to delineate the content and tasks included in its tests. Content Guidelines for the HT and HTL examinations appear in Chapter 7, "Examination Content Guidelines."

It will be helpful to scan major journals to keep up with the innovations in the field. Textbooks may be updated only every few years, whereas new questions are added to the examinations every examination cycle. Therefore, it is possible that questions will be asked on content that is not yet in textbooks but has been added to the literature via journals and other periodicals.

Get Enough Rest Before the Examination

Ease up on your studying before the examination. Try to get plenty of rest and eat a light meal before going to take the examination. The HT and HTL examinations take two-and-a-half hours.

Locate the Test Center

Plan to arrive at the test site a half hour before your scheduled appointment to check in and familiarize yourself with the area. **You must present a picture ID and the admission letter before you will be admitted to the test.**

Chapter 5

Taking the Examination by Computer

Introduction

The Board of Registry has thoroughly studied computerized adaptive testing. Results of this in-depth assessment demonstrate clearly that computerized adaptive tests are more reliable than traditional written tests in measuring ability and reaching a pass-fail decision for certification. Candidates have the same opportunity to demonstrate the required level of knowledge and skill to achieve certification on a computerized test as on a written examination.

Advantages

Computerized adaptive testing offers many advantages over written examinations:
1) testing is by individual appointment in a comfortable computer carrel which affords quiet and privacy for the candidate;
2) candidates are required to answer fewer questions;
3) less time is required to take the test;
4) it is simpler to enter answers on the computer keyboard than to record answers on a separate answer sheet; and
5) score reporting requires a shorter time (10 days).

Prior knowledge of computer use is not required. The candidate answers each question by pressing the number key; 1,2,3, or 4, corresponding to the answer number selected. Candidates may also use the computer mouse to choose and record answers. Pressing the ENTER key records the response. There is also a HELP screen that permits the candidate to review the instructions on how to enter responses.

Both the HT and the HTL exams consist of 100 questions. The total time allowed for each exam is 2.5 hours.

Test Center Procedures

1) Scratch paper will be provided for you. No books, dictionaries, or paper may be taken into the examination room.

2) The Board of Registry allows the use of nonprogrammable calculators during the test. They must be brought into the testing site without carrying cases.

3) You must bring photo identification and the admission letter (sent to you after your examination eligibility has been determined) to the test center.

4) You will be required to acknowledge the following statement: "I have read the Examination Instructions. I understand that if an applicant is caught cheating on a certifying examination, his/her results will be held until such time as the applicant appeals to the Board of Registry, at which time the Board will decide each individual case. I certify that I am the candidate whose social security number appeared on the first screen. I also certify that, because of the confidential nature of these copyright materials, I will not retain or copy any examination materials and I will not otherwise reveal the content of these materials." By pressing ENTER you agree to the above statement and your examination will begin.

Irregularities

If an examinee is discovered engaging in inappropriate conduct during the examination, such as looking at notes or otherwise giving or obtaining unauthorized information or aid, the test center personnel will immediately notify the Board of Registry office in writing. Inappropriate conduct by an examinee may result in invalidation of the examinee's test results, as well as revocation of current certification and a bar of admission to Board of Registry-sponsored examinations in the future. Other appropriate action may also be taken against the examinee.

Suggestions for Taking the Test

1) Read the instructions carefully before beginning. A HELP screen that reviews the instructions is available at any time during the test.

2) Read the questions carefully, looking for words such as "best," "most likely," "least likely," and "not."

3) Read all the answer choices before answering. Sometimes what appears initially to be a correct answer may not be the **best** answer.

4) Budget your time so you can answer each question. Do not spend an inordinate amount of time on any one question.

5) Answer each question to the best of your ability when it is presented. There is no extra penalty for guessing on Board of Registry examinations. In other words, if you have some knowledge about the content of the question, select the best response. The computer requires that you answer each question as it is presented before you can proceed to another question.

6) Record your answer by pressing the number key that corresponds to your answer choice and then pressing ENTER. You may change your answer as often as you wish before you press ENTER. You may also use the computer mouse to select and record your answer.

7) Try to stay relaxed so that you can think through clearly and logically the problems presented on the examination.

8) After all questions have been answered, directions for reviewing the test and changing responses will appear on the screen. You may review your answers for some or all questions at the end of the test. The response you previously selected appears highlighted. You may choose to change the response by pressing the key for a different response number. By pressing the ENTER key, you record your newly selected response and move to the next question. But think carefully before altering a response.

9) Upon completing your review, press the "Q" (QUIT) key, followed by the ENTER key, to end the test. A message indicating that the answers are being recorded then appears on the screen and the test is complete.

Chapter 6

Examination Development

Examination Committee

The Histotechnology Examination Committee prepares the histotechnologist and histologic technician examinations and is composed of histotechnologists, histologic technicians, and pathologists. The committee represents both diverse geographical areas and diverse types of practice. The responsibility of item writing, evaluation, and selection rests with the examination committee members. Question writing requires mastery of the subject as well as an understanding of the examination population and mastery of written communication skills. Question review by the entire committee ensures that the item adheres to appropriate technical and/or scientific principles. The committee is also responsible for maintaining the currency of the content of the examinations. It is supported by the Board of Registry staff, which provides expertise in psychometrics and examination development.

Criterion-Referenced Testing

The Board of Registry's process of examination development and analysis is based on the concept of criterion-referenced testing. Generally, a criterion-referenced examination is designed to ascertain an individual's knowledge as measured with respect to a set of previously defined competencies that summarize the domain of knowledge and skill represented on the examination. Each examination question is designed to test some aspect of the competencies that have been developed as criteria against which examinees are measured. Thus, every question on an examination becomes a "criterion" against which the examinee is measured. If an examinee answers an item correctly, he or she has met the criterion; if an examinee answers incorrectly, he or she has not met the criterion. Because it is unlikely that one question would be the absolute measure of a competency, the Board of Registry examinations are carefully planned so that multiple questions measure competencies.

In criterion-referenced testing, the domain of practice of the histotechnologist or histologic technician is delineated in competency statements and content outlines (see Chapter 7, "Examination Content Guidelines"). These competency statements serve as the basis for the examination questions.

Purpose of the Examination

The Board of Registry certification examinations measure an examinee's level of skill and knowledge (competency) at a particular point in time. Each examination question, because it is tied to a competency statement, contributes to the pass/fail decision. Because questions must accurately distinguish between qualified and unqualified candidates, each question is carefully written, reviewed, and evaluated. A very comprehensive process is used to assure that each question measures what it is intended to measure.

Components of Competency

Examination items are written from competency statements. The 3 components of competence tested are (1) knowledge, (2) technical skill, and (3) cognitive skill. The components expand into competency statements in which knowledge is represented by the content areas and technical skill is represented by task and task definitions (see Chapter 7).

Knowledge
This is the first dimension of competency and a criterion against which examinees are measured. Knowledge is the content base upon which the field of practice in histotechnology is built. Content areas of histotechnology typically include fixation, processing, microtomy, staining, and laboratory operations.

Technical Skill
The second component of competency and a criterion against which the examinee is measured may be defined as the ability to complete an assigned activity or apply knowledge to a procedure. The implication is that laboratory tasks can be defined and that one's ability to perform them can be measured on a test. While these are not the only tasks completed by laboratory staff, they are the areas that are considered essential to test on during the examination.

Cognitive Skill
The third component of competence is the ability to deal with data at various cognitive skill levels. *Cognitive skill* refers to the cognitive or mental processes required to answer the question. Questions are classified into 3 cognitive skill levels, based on the structure of the question. The 3 cognitive skill levels used by the Board of Registry are defined as follows:

Recall (level 1),
> the ability to recall or recognize previously learned (memorized) knowledge ranging from specific facts to complete theories;

Interpretive skills (level 2),
> the ability to use recalled knowledge to interpret or apply verbal, numeric, or visual data;

Problem solving (level 3)
> the ability to use recalled knowledge and the interpretation/application of distinct criteria to resolve a problem or situation and/or make an appropriate decision.

The cognitive skill level of a question is influenced by the construction of the stem in concert with the responses. Thus, a concept such as immunofluorescence provides the content for the development of questions on all 3 cognitive skill levels. All items appearing on a Board of Registry examination were written to test one of the competency statements listed in Chapter 7.

Question Development

The Board of Registry examinations consist of multiple-choice questions. A multiple-choice question may be defined as a measuring device that contains a *stem* and 4 *responses*, one of which is the best answer. The form is flexible so that an item may ask a specific question, describe a situation, or report laboratory results, etc.

The stem of a multiple choice question

1) asks a question,
2) gives an incomplete statement,
3) states an issue, or
4) describes a situation

The content of the stem is designed to focus on a central theme or problem, using clear and precise language, without excessive length that can confuse or distract examinees. The stem may describe clinical data and laboratory results that require interpretation or problem solving. The question or issue presented in the stem is relevant to the knowledge and task delineated in a competency statement.

The 4 responses present the "best" answer and the "distractors." Each multiple-choice question has 4 independent responses. The best answer is the one agreed upon by the experts; however, the other 3 distractors may seem plausible to an examinee who has partial, incomplete, or inappropriate knowledge. The distractors may therefore be considered logical misconceptions of the best answer. The responses are written to be parallel in content, length, and category of information.

As you review the questions included in this book, it may be useful to note the construction of the question carefully, reviewing both the stem and responses as you practice selecting the best answer.

Color Plates and Other Visual Materials

Some of the questions on the examination will refer to color photographs of clinical materials or other visual materials such as graphs or charts. All subject areas may have color photographs. Color photographs are also provided in this book. You may wish to study other books containing color plates (often called atlases) as you prepare for this part of the examination. Some of these books are listed in the reading lists at the end of this book. In addition, many journals frequently contain photographs and graphs. Examples are *Laboratory Medicine*, a monthly journal of the American Society of Clinical Pathologists, and the *Journal of Histotechnology*, a quarterly journal of the National Society of Histotechnology. These and other journals may be available in the laboratory or a medical library as well as by subscription.

To sharpen your ability to understand and analyze visual materials, a good exercise might be to look at an illustration and attempt to evaluate it without referring to the legend. Once you have analyzed the photograph, compare your analysis with the legend. Practice this exercise in your reading whenever the article or book contains photographic material.

Preparation of Examinations

The Board of Registry maintains databases containing more than 10,000 examination questions. These computerized databases have extensive identification and sorting capabilities. The number of multiple choice questions in each computerized histologic technician or histotechnologist examination is 100.

Board of Registry examinations are carefully developed according to the specifications of the content guidelines. Each examination is constructed according to a "multidimensional examination blueprint." A computer algorithm implements these criteria for each examination. Although different questions may be presented to individual examinees, the overall content distribution will match the test specifications delineated in the content guidelines.

Chapter 7

Examination Content Guidelines

The content of each examination is determined by the competency statements and content outlines developed and published by the Board of Registry. These competency statements and content outlines are provided to show the topics that will be covered on the examinations. The most current content guidelines can be found on the Internet at www.ascp.org/bor/certification.

*With regard to Laboratory Operations and the performance of basic, existing laboratory procedures involving Fixation, Processing/Embedding, Microtomy and Staining at career entry, the **Histologic Technician***:

DEFINES OR IDENTIFIES PRINCIPLES OF
Methods
Terminology
Reactions and results
Sources of error
Anatomy, histology, physiology, biochemistry, and pathology
Standard operating procedures of methods and instrumentation

SELECTS OR PREPARES APPROPRIATE
Methods
Procedural courses of action
Reagents
Instruments
Controls

CALCULATES RESULTS

CORRELATES REACTIONS OR RESULTS OF BASIC AND SPECIAL METHODS
With histology to access procedures

EVALUATES REACTIONS, RESULTS, METHODS TO
Verify results
Check for common problems
Check for potential sources of error
Take predetermined corrective action

With regard to Laboratory Operations and the performance of basic and special laboratory procedures involving Fixation, Processing/Embedding, Microtomy, and Staining at career entry, the **Histotechnologist:**

DEFINES OR IDENTIFIES PRINCIPLES OF
Methods
Terminology
Reactions and results
Sources of error
Anatomy, histology, physiology, biochemistry, and pathology
Standard operating procedures of methods and instrumentation
Management and education

SELECTS OR PREPARES APPROPRIATE
Methods
Procedural courses of action
Reagents
Instruments
Controls

CALCULATES RESULTS

CORRELATES REACTIONS OR RESULTS OF BASIC AND SPECIAL METHODS
With anatomy, histology, physiology, biochemistry, or pathology to assess procedures

EVALUATES REACTIONS, RESULTS, METHODS TO
Assist in ascertaining disease states
Check for common and unusual problems
Take corrective action
Verify quality control
Assess validity
Assure laboratory safety
Check for potential sources of error

CONTENT OUTLINE
HISTOLOGIC TECHNICIAN HT(ASCP) AND HISTOTECNOLOGIST HTL (ASCP)

I. FIXATION (10% to 25%)

A. Tissues
1. Morphology/Anatomy
2. Cell/Component preservation
3. Pathology*
4. Biochemistry principles/theories*

B. Procedures
1. Light microscopy
2. Electron microscopy
3. Special stains
4. Frozen sections/tissues
5. Enzyme histochemistry
6. Immunohistochemistry
7. Artifacts/Precipitates/Pigments
8. Quality control
9. Cytologic specimens

C. Parameters
1. Size of specimen
2. Volume of specimen/fixative
3. Time of fixation
4. Temperature of specimen/fixative
5. Other

D. Reagents
1. Types/Components
2. Properties/Functions/Actions
3. Quality control
4. Chemistry principles/theories*

E. Instrumentation (eg, microwave)
1. Components
2. Use
3. Maintenance
4. Troubleshooting
5. Quality control

II. PROCESSING/EMBEDDING (10% to 14%)

A. Tissues
1. Morphology/Anatomy
2. Cell/Component preservation

B. Procedures
1. Light microscopy
2. Frozen sections/tissues
3. Enzyme histochemistry
4. Calcified/Decalcified tissue
5. Immunohistochemistry
6. Quality control
7. Cytologic specimens

C. Instrumentation
1. Components
2. Use
3. Maintenance
4. Troubleshooting
5. Quality control

D. Reagents
1. Types/Components
2. Properties/Function/Action
3. Quality control
4. Chemistry principles/theories*

III. MICROTOMY (10% to 14%)

A. Tissues
1. Morphology/Anatomy
2. Cell/Component demonstration

B. Procedures
1. Paraffin
2. Frozen Section
3. Agar/gelatin
4. Quality control
5. Glycol methacrylate*

C. Instrumentation
1. Components
2. Use
3. Maintenance
4. Troubleshooting
5. Quality control

IV. STAINING (40% to 50%)

A. Tissues
1. Morphology/Anatomy
2. Cell/Component demonstration
3. Function
4. Pathology*
5. Biochemistry principles/theories*

B. Procedures
1. Nucleus/Cytoplasm (eg, H&E)
2. Blood/Bone marrow
3. Carbohydrates
4. Connective/Supporting tissue
5. Lipids
6. Microorganisms
7. Nerve
8. Pigments/Minerals/Granules
9. Quality control

C. Miscellaneous Procedures
1. Nucleic acids
2. Tissues/Cells/Components (eg, fibrin, mast cells)
3. Quality control
4. Enzymes*
5. Immunohistochemistry*

D. Instrumentation
1. Components
2. Use
3. Maintenance
4. Troubleshooting
5. Quality control

E. Reagents/Dyes
1. Types/Components
2. Properties/Functions/Actions
3. Quality control
4. Chemistry principles/theories*

F. Mounting Procedures
1. Media
2. Cover glass
3. Refractive index*

V. LABORATORY OPERATIONS (10% to 15%)

A. Safety
1. Storage
2. Disposal
3. Hazards
4. Regulations
5. Procedures
6. Quality control

B. Laboratory Mathematics
1. Metric system
2. Percent solutions/Dilutions
3. Normal/Molar solutions

C. Ancillary Equipment/Instruments, (eg, microwave, computers, pH meter, solvent recovery)
1. Components
2. Use
3. Maintenance
4. Troubleshooting
5. Quality control

D. Management*
1. Theories*
2. Procedures*

E. Education*
1. Theories*
2. Procedures*

F. Regulations*
1. Federal government*
2. Accrediting agencies*

*HTL EXAMINATION ONLY

All Board of Registry examinations use conventional units for results and reference ranges.

Chapter 8

Examination Scoring

Criterion-referenced testing is a form of measurement designed to measure an examinee's performance compared with an established standard or criterion. For the Board of Registry examinations, this criterion is called the *minimum pass score* (MPS). Any individual who achieves the level of performance represented by the minimum pass score passes the examination. Those who do not meet this standard fail the examination.

In 1980, the Board of Registry adopted a policy of criterion-referenced testing. Absolute standards are established by the Examination Committee through a systematic evaluation of the content and skill represented in each question. The standard was established as a scaled score of 400. All examinations are equated to this standard. This ensures that all candidates meet the same standard regardless of the difficulty of the particular group of questions posed to a candidate.

Question Development and Analysis

The Board of Registry uses standard procedures for psychometric analysis to ensure that each examinee receives a fair examination.

Examination questions are evaluated through item analysis statistics. These statistics are used to identify unacceptable items. To ensure the continued quality of the examinations, questions are reviewed periodically and those found to be unsatisfactory are excluded from the examination item pool.

Item statistical analysis includes traditional item analysis and item response theory (IRT) analysis. The Rasch model is used for the IRT analysis. Both approaches to analysis include an assessment of item difficulty. Difficulty correlates with the percentage of examinees selecting each response. The correct response or best answer should draw the highest proportion of the population, while the distractors should draw a smaller percentage of the population. This provides an index of how easy or difficult the question was for a particular population. IRT analysis then translates the percentage into an absolute log-odds unit of difficulty, so that the relative difficulty of items can be monitored across tests.

In traditional item analysis, the concept of *discrimination* provides an indication of how well the question differentiates between those examinees who did well on the total examination and those who did not. The computation compares or correlates the performance of candidates who selected the best answer on the question with the performance of those candidates who did well on the total examination. A positive correlation is anticipated for the correct response (best answer), and negative correlations are anticipated for the distractors. This is based on the assumption that those who did well on the question should do well on the test.

IRT analysis provides a *fit statistic*, which is an assessment of how well the item fits the expectations of the Rasch model. The basic expectation is that examinees who are more able will answer any item correctly more frequently than examinees who are less able. Another expectation is that easier items will be answered correctly by more examinees than harder items. When these 2 relatively simple expectations are not met, the "fit statistic" flags the question for review.

Each HT and HTL practical examination is graded by 3 slide graders. To allow for differences in the levels of severity of each grader, the Rasch model is extended to include a facet for graders. The probability equation is also extended to include the influence of the graders' severity. Thus the potential bias of any grader is accounted for before examinees' scores are calculated, and all examinees are scored comparably and fairly.

Score Reporting

Examinee Performance Reports are generated and distributed to the examinees within 10 days following the date on which the computerized exam was taken. (Test results are not released by telephone to anyone.) The purpose of the report is to provide examinees with information about their performance on the examination.

The following explanation refers to the sample Examinee Performance Reports in Figures 1 – 3. The first paragraph provides an explanation of how to interpret the profile. Key information is presented under "YOUR PERFORMANCE SUMMARY." A scaled minimum pass score (MPS) of 400 is the required passing score. Individuals who achieve or exceed the MPS pass the examination; others fail. The decision to pass or fail is based on the candidate ability measure for the total test. Pass or fail status is noted under STATUS.

Figure 1 shows a performance report for a candidate who passed. **Figure 2** shows a report for a candidate who failed. Subtest scaled scores for Fixation (FIXT), Laboratory Operations (LO), Microtomy (MICR), Processing/Embedding (PROC), and Staining (ST) are included in this report (but not in passing reports). These subtest scores provide the failing candidate with information concerning strengths and weaknesses which may be useful for future study.

Figure 3 shows a performance report for a candidate who failed the practical portion for the HT/HTL certification examination. **Figure 4** shows a combined performance report. This report shows both the computer-adaptive test (CAT) and the practical portions of the HT/HTL certification examination.

Figure 1: Sample of Examinee Performance Report–Pass

EXAMINEE PERFORMANCE REPORT

000-00-0000   HT(ASCP) 00000
JOHN DOE
123 MAIN STREET
ANYWHERE, USA

THIS REPORT PROVIDES INFORMATION CONCERNING YOUR EXAMINATION
PERFORMANCE. A SCALED MINIMUM PASS SCORE (MPS) OF 400 ON THE
TOTAL TEST WAS REQUIRED TO PASS.

YOUR PERFORMANCE SUMMARY FOR THE TOTAL HT EXAMINATION TAKEN
ON 03/03/1993:

MPS	YOUR SCORE	STATUS
400	514	PASS

Figure 2: Sample of Examinee Performance Report—Fail

EXAMINEE PERFORMANCE REPORT

000-00-0000
JANE DOE
246 MAIN STRET
ANYWHERE, USA

THIS REPORT PROVIDES INFORMATION CONCERNING YOUR EXAMINATION PERFORMANCE. A SCALED MINIMUM PASS SCORE (MPS) OF 400 ON THE TOTAL TEST WAS REQUIRED TO PASS.

YOUR PERFORMANCE SUMMARY FOR THE TOTAL HTL EXAMINATION TAKEN ON 03/12/1993:

MPS	YOUR SCORE	STATUS
400	318	FAIL

SUBTEST PERFORMANCE SUMMARY

SUBTESTS	[PERCENT OF TOTAL TEST]	SCALED SCORES
FIXATION	[25%]	334
LABORATORY OPERATIONS	[15%]	336
MICROTOMY	[10%]	331
PROCESSING/EMBEDDING	[10%]	291
STAINING	[40%]	299

Figure 3: Sample of Practical Examinee Performance Report

HT PRACTICAL EXAMINEE PERFORMANCE REPORT
****

000-00-0000
JANE DOE   AUGUST, 1993

MPS: 400   SCORE: 350   STATUS: FAIL
****

TO ASSIST YOU IN EVALUATING YOUR PERFORMANCE, THE COMMENTS ASSOCIATED WITH THE SCORE YOU WERE AWARDED ARE INDICATED FOR EACH SLIDE. IF NO COMMENT IS RECORDED, YOU EARNED A PERFECT SCORE ON THAT SLIDE. PLEASE REFER TO THE PRACTICAL BOOKLET FOR THE KEY TO THE COMMENT LETTERS.

BASELINE PERFORMANCE

TISSUE/STAIN	BLOCKS	LAB/COV	FIX/PRO	MICRO	STAIN	LABEL	SIZE
UTERUS H&E	a		b	b	b		a
BREAST H&E							
LIVER H&E	****		e	c			
PANCREAS H&E	f	e				a	
AORTA H&E	b						
SM INTEST H&E	****						
CERVIX H&E	****			f			
BONE H&E					y		
SKIN H&E				h			
MED/SP CRD H&E	****	e					
SPLEEN IRON				c			
KIDNEY PASH		e			C		
LYMPH RETIC							
AFB CRB FUCHSIN	****	e					
FUNGUS GMS	****	e			E		

**** = BLOCK NOT GRADED

26

Figure 4: Sample of Combined Examinee Performance Report

EXAMINEE PERFORMANCE REPORT SUMMARY

HISTOLOGIC TECHNICIAN EXAMINATION

000-00-0000   HT(ASCP)   99999
JOHN DOE
123 USA STREET
ANYWHERE, USA

THIS REPORT PROVIDES INFORMATION CONCERNING YOUR EXAMINATION
PERFORMANCE. A SCALED MINIMUM PASS SCORE (MPS) OF 400 ON THE
TOTAL TEST WAS REQUIRED TO PASS.

YOUR PERFORMANCE SUMMARY FOR THE TOTAL HT EXAMINATION APPEARS
IN THE TABLE BELOW.

	MPS	EXAM DATE	YOUR SCORE	STATUS
MCQ	400	09/15/1993	450	PASS
PRC	400	08/01/1993	509	PASS

TOTAL EXAMINATION   PASS

Chapter 9

Fixation

The following items have been identified as appropriate for both entry level histologic technicians and histotechnologists.

1. An example of an additive fixative is one that contains:

   a. mercuric chloride
   b. acetic acid
   c. ethyl alcohol
   d. acetone

2. When compared with tissue fixed in formalin, tissue fixed in zinc-formalin will show:

   a. better ultrastructural preservation
   b. decreased immunoreactivity
   c. increased enzyme activity
   d. superior nuclear detail

3. Microscopic examination of an H&E-stained section fixed in formalin shows marked nuclear bubbling. One most often sees this artifact if the specimen is processed following:

   a. underfixation
   b. prolonged fixation
   c. microwave fixation
   d. frozen sectioning

4. Microscopic evaluation of H&E-stained sections from a surgically removed small bowel specimen show an absence of much of the epithelium in otherwise normal tissue. This most likely resulted from:

   a. mechanical trauma
   b. delayed fixation
   c. ulceration
   d. poor choice of fixative

5. A specimen of kidney must be shipped to another city for immunofluorescence studies. The specimen should be placed in:

   a. saline
   b. Michel solution
   c. buffered formalin
   d. Orth solution

6. In a certain project it is important to use a fixative that contains acetic acid yet stabilizes erythrocyte membranes. One fixative that could be used is:

   a. Zenker solution
   b. Bouin solution
   c. Gendre solution
   d. Hollande solution

7. When a microwave oven is used for fixation, the most critical factor is the:

   a. preparation of the formalin solution
   b. use of glass containers
   c. control of the temperature
   d. osmolality of the fixation solution

8. To adequately remove the calcium in a specimen containing areas of microcalcification, the tissue could be fixed in:

   a. Hollande solution
   b. neutral buffered formalin
   c. B-5 solution
   d. Zamboni solution

9. Which of the following fixatives contains copper acetate?

   a. Hollande
   b. Bouin
   c. Gendre
   d. Zamboni

10. A specimen is submitted with the statement that it was fixed in formalin. Microscopic sections show marked lysis of erythrocytes. This indicates that the fixative most likely was:

    a. prepared with too much formalin
    b. buffered above neutrality
    c. acetified with acetic acid
    d. not formalin

11. Fixatives are classified as additive because of the:

    a. addition of several chemicals to the solution
    b. addition, or binding of the fixative, to tissue proteins
    c. additional reactions occurring with longer fixation
    d. additional reactive tissue sites available for dye binding

12. The only kidney biopsy tissue available has been fixed in phosphate-buffered glutaraldehyde for 2 hours and then placed in phosphate buffer solution. If a portion of this tissue is processed for light microscopy, sections would most likely show:

   a. very poor glomerular preservation
   b. decreased uptake of hematoxylin
   c. lysis of cytoplasmic elements
   d. nonspecific PAS staining

13. Uric acid crystals are preserved only when tissue is fixed in:

   a. absolute alcohol
   b. neutral buffered formalin
   c. Orth solution
   d. Zamboni solution

14. Improper preservation of tissue will result if there is:

   a. a delay in fixation
   b. rapid penetration of the fixing fluid
   c. prolonged storage following formalin fixation
   d. rapid dehydration, clearing, embedding, and sectioning

15. A good fixative will:

   a. render cell constituents soluble
   b. minimize differences in tissue refractive indices
   c. protect tissue against alteration by subsequent processing
   d. minimally affect tissue metabolic processes

16. The function of methanol in commercial formalin solutions is to:

   a. retard the polymerization of formaldehyde
   b. prevent the formation of formic acid
   c. stabilize the formalin at a basic pH
   d. permit the storage of formalin at room temperature

17. The subsequent demonstration of chromaffin granules requires which of the following fixatives?

   a. Orth
   b. Bouin
   c. B-5
   d. formalin

18. In electron microscopy, Zamboni fluid, glutaraldehyde, and osmium tetroxide function as:

   a. dehydrating agents
   b. clearing agents
   c. embedding media
   d. fixatives

19. Tissue will remain unfixed if placed in:

   a. potassium dichromate
   b. sodium borate
   c. osmium tetroxide
   d. zinc chloride

20. Bouin solution is contraindicated for:

   a. small tissue biopsies
   b. tissue intended for subsequent trichrome stains
   c. tissue to be stained by the Feulgen reaction
   d. routine tissue sections

21. Formalin pigment can be removed from tissue sections by treatment with 10%:

   a. hydrochloric acid in 70% alcohol
   b. nitric acid in 70% alcohol
   c. sulfuric acid in 70% alcohol
   d. ammonium hydroxide in 70% alcohol

22. Stock neutralized formalin is prepared in the laboratory by storing the solution over a layer of calcium carbonate. The solution withdrawn from this stock container will:

   a. become acidic
   b. become alkaline
   c. remain neutral
   d. exhibit metachromasia

23. Microscopic evaluation reveals a very poorly-stained H&E section of spleen. These results will be difficult to remedy if the problem is:

   a. poor fixation
   b. improper sectioning
   c. poor staining
   d. incorrect section placement

24. To make a 10% formalin solution, how many mL of water should be added to 300 mL of 37% to 40% formaldehyde solution?

   a. 1800
   b. 2500
   c. 2700
   d. 3600

25. One action of acetic acid is to:

   a. exert a shrinking effect on tissue
   b. render nucleoprotein acidophilic
   c. form salt linkages between protein chains
   d. coagulate nucleoproteins

26. Aldehyde fixatives are used for electron microscopy preparations because they:

   a. are readily available
   b. visibly stain tissue
   c. preserve cell ultrastructure
   d. coagulate tissue lipids

27. A fixative containing potassium dichromate:

   a. is suitable when histochemical techniques are planned
   b. will result in excellent subsequent silver staining
   c. is preferred for the preservation of argentaffin cells
   d. will make tissue more receptive to eosin staining

28. If mercuric chloride is used alone for fixation, it will:

   a. leave tissue proteins uncoagulated
   b. produce a very acidic solution
   c. penetrate poorly and cause excessive shrinkage
   d. decrease tissue affinity for stains

29. Tissue stored for long periods of time in unbuffered formalin or in acetate-buffered formalin may show brown, crystalline pigment in stained sections. To remove this pigment prior to staining it is necessary to treat the section in:

   a. saturated alcoholic picric acid
   b. alcoholic lithium chloride
   c. iodine and sodium thiosulfate
   d. potassium permanganate and oxalic acid

30. For good fixation of specimens for electron microscopy, it is recommended that the tissue segment be no larger than:

   a. 1 mm^3
   b. 2 mm^3
   c. 1 cm^3
   d. 2 cm^3

31. Waxes that are commonly used in the preparation of tissue sections for light microscopic evaluation are NOT used in electron microscopy because tissues prepared in wax:

   a. cannot be stained with osmium tetroxide
   b. are too hard for thin sectioning
   c. are not transparent
   d. will not withstand an electron beam

32. Following fixation with Bouin solution, tissue should be washed with:

   a. absolute alcohol
   b. 50% to 70% alcohol
   c. 20% to 40% alcohol
   d. saline solution

33. Zenker fluid is the recommended fixative for subsequent:

    a. PTAH staining
    b. frozen sectioning
    c. hemosiderin preservation
    d. erythrocyte demonstration

34. The acetic acid present in some fixatives:

    a. coagulates and shrinks cytoplasmic proteins
    b. dissolves some cytoplasmic organelles and deposits
    c. penetrates tissue very slowly and incompletely
    d. hardens the tissue markedly

35. Absolute ethanol is a poor choice for the fixation of:

    a. glycogen
    b. pigments
    c. lipids
    d. blood smears

36. Which of the following fixatives may give false-positive results in carbohydrate demonstration?

    a. neutral buffered formalin
    b. Bouin solution
    c. Gendre solution
    d. glutaraldehyde

37. It is necessary to adjust the pH of most formalin solutions because of the presence of:

    a. methanol
    b. formic acid
    c. paraformaldehyde
    d. carbon dioxide

38. The rate of fixation varies with the fixative and is also dependent upon the:

    a. grossing pathologist's preference
    b. expected completion time of the report
    c. anticipated special stains
    d. temperature of the fixative

39. Carnoy solution is recommended for the preservation of:

    a. acid-fast bacilli
    b. nucleic acids
    c. lipids
    d. red blood cells

40. Orth solution contains all of the following EXCEPT:

   a. potassium dichromate
   b. mercuric chloride
   c. sodium sulfate
   d. 37% to 40% formaldehyde

41. Formalin pigment is generally created in tissues fixed in formalin when the pH:

   a. rises above 6
   b. falls below 6
   c. is buffered to neutrality
   d. is 7.2

42. A universal fixative used for routine purposes that allows a broad spectrum of staining procedures is:

   a. Zenker fluid
   b. Zamboni PAF
   c. 10% neutral buffered formalin
   d. Carnoy solution

43. One advantage of fixing tissue in Zenker solution is that:

   a. the prolonged treatment keeps the tissue soft and pliable
   b. Zenker-fixed tissues stain brilliantly
   c. artifactual pigments are not formed
   d. washing after fixation is not required

44. A tissue section was not initially placed in the fixative required for a staining procedure. However, after deparaffinization and rehydration, sections frequently can be stained anyway if they are:

   a. soaked in a solution of lithium carbonate prior to staining
   b. revitalized by washing in a solution of sodium bisulfite
   c. post-fixed in the appropriate fixative prior to staining
   d. treated with hydrogen peroxide

45. Helly fluid contains all of the following EXCEPT:

   a. mercuric chloride
   b. potassium dichromate
   c. sodium sulfate
   d. glacial acetic acid

46. Fixation in Bouin solution is:

   a. recommended for the Feulgen reaction
   b. excellent for ultrastructural preservation
   c. the cause of considerable swelling of tissue
   d. frequently used for endocrine tissues

47. B-5 fixative contains:

    a. mercuric chloride, sodium acetate, and glacial acetic acid
    b. mercuric chloride, potassium dichromate, and glacial acetic acid
    c. mercuric chloride, sodium acetate, and 37% to 40% formaldehyde
    d. mercuric chloride, potassium dichromate, and 37% to 40% formaldehyde

48. Pigment caused by mercury-containing fixatives can be removed from tissues by:

    a. saturated alcoholic picric acid
    b. iodine-sodium thiosulfate
    c. washing in running water
    d. potassium hydroxide in water

49. Which of the following fixatives has a mordanting effect on tissue?

    a. Carnoy solution
    b. 10% calcium formalin
    c. absolute alcohol
    d. Zenker solution

50. Tissue should be placed in a suitable fixative immediately after removal from the body to:

    a. prevent decomposition due to enzymatic activity
    b. permit the dehydrant to function properly
    c. inhibit cross-linking of tissue proteins
    d. stabilize tissue carbohydrates

51. Baker calcium-formalin fixative is recommended for the best preservation and subsequent demonstration of:

    a. glycogen
    b. phospholipids
    c. amyloid
    d. estrogen receptors

52. For most fixatives, the volume of fixing fluid in relation to the volume of tissue should be:

    a. 2 to 5 times
    b. 6 to 9 times
    c. 10 to 14 times
    d. 15 to 20 times

53. Ultrastructural preservation will be very poor following fixation in:

    a. Zamboni PAF
    b. 2% buffered glutaraldehyde
    c. osmium tetroxide
    d. 10% aqueous formalin

54. The fixation of tissue begins at the:

   a. center and proceeds outward
   b. center and proceeds inward
   c. periphery and proceeds outward
   d. periphery and proceeds inward

55. Zinc-formalin fixatives:

   a. give poor ultrastructural preservation
   b. can be used to preserve enzymes
   c. result in poor nuclear detail
   d. will not coagulate tissue proteins

56. Zamboni PAF refers to a fixative containing:

   a. potassium dichromate, acetic acid, and formaldehyde
   b. potassium aluminum sulfate and paraformaldehyde
   c. buffered picric acid and formaldehyde
   d. picric acid, acetic acid, and formaldehyde

57. Excess fixative must be removed from specimens before placing them in dehydrating solutions if the fixative contains:

   a. glutaraldehyde
   b. mercuric chloride
   c. picric acid
   d. potassium dichromate

58. The preferred fixative when tissue is to be stained for the presence of simple fats is:

   a. Zenker
   b. Helly
   c. Hollande
   d. neutral buffered formalin

59. Which of the following is recommended for central nervous system tissues to be stained with the Cajal technique?

   a. neutralized formalin
   b. formalin ammonium bromide
   c. paraformaldehyde
   d. alcoholic formalin

60. When osmium tetroxide is used as a fixative in histology, it:

   a. destroys lipids
   b. interferes with staining
   c. leaves tissue very soft
   d. distorts cell membranes

61. The breakdown of tissue due to enzyme activity is called:

    a. polymerization
    b. putrefaction
    c. autolysis
    d. osmosis

62. The fixative of choice for the demonstration of urate crystals is:

    a. neutral buffered formalin
    b. absolute alcohol
    c. Bouin solution
    d. Zenker solution

63. A good fixative for routine use is one that:

    a. makes tissue more permeable to fluids
    b. is hypotonic to the tissue constituents
    c. enhances putrefaction of tissue components
    d. promotes tissue autolysis

64. A pigment caused by chromate-containing fixatives can be prevented by treating the tissue prior to processing with:

    a. running water
    b. iodine
    c. picric acid
    d. potassium permanganate

65. When fixing tissue with formaldehyde or glutaraldehyde, proper enzyme activity and preservation of structure depend upon all of the following EXCEPT:

    a. pH
    b. time and temperature
    c. concentration and purity of the reagent
    d. type of tissue

66. Formic acid present in commercial formalin solutions may:

    a. facilitate pigment formation
    b. precipitate hemosiderin
    c. promote staining
    d. cause tissue shrinkage

67. Carnoy solution is a combination of which of the following chemicals?

    a. absolute alcohol, acetone, and glacial acetic acid
    b. cedarwood oil, absolute alcohol, and glacial acetic acid
    c. acetone, chloroform, and absolute alcohol
    d. chloroform, glacial acetic acid, and absolute alcohol

68. When staining chromaffin cells for the diagnosis of pheochromocytoma, it is necessary to fix the tissue in a:

    a. mercury fixative
    b. primary chromate fixative
    c. formalin fixative
    d. picric acid fixative

69. When liver tissue is fixed with 2% to 3% glutaraldehyde:

    a. protein is only partially preserved
    b. the penetration rate is very rapid
    c. a chemical reaction occurs with lipids
    d. the ultrastructure is preserved

70. A poor fixative is characterized by:

    a. the absence of shrinking or swelling of tissue
    b. inactivation of tissue enzymes
    c. slow tissue penetration
    d. the absence of distortion or dissolution

71. Which of the following fixatives requires washing with water before processing?

    a. Carnoy
    b. Bouin
    c. 10% formalin
    d. Zenker

72. Bouin solution contains all of the following EXCEPT:

    a. picric acid
    b. absolute alcohol
    c. 37% to 40% formaldehyde
    d. glacial acetic acid

73. Coagulant fixatives:

    a. change the spongework of proteins into meshes
    b. produce fewer artifacts than noncoagulant fixatives
    c. act very slowly to fix tissues
    d. leave protein linkages unaffected

74. The breakdown of tissue by bacterial action is called:

    a. autolysis
    b. putrefaction
    c. denaturation
    d. oxidation

75. When ultrastructural preservation is of the utmost importance, the fixative used should have a pH of:

   a. 6.8 to 7.0
   b. 7.2 to 7.4
   c. 7.6 to 7.8
   d. 8.0 to 8.2

76. A fixative that produces a diffuse brownish black pigment is:

   a. Bouin
   b. Carnoy
   c. Zenker
   d. alcohol

77. For the BEST preservation of staining properties during long-term storage, tissues should be stored in:

   a. buffered formalin
   b. 10% formal-saline
   c. 70% ethanol
   d. Zamboni solution

78. Ethanol is useful as a fixative because it:

   a. rapidly dehydrates tissue
   b. increases tissue basophilia
   c. stabilizes red cell membranes
   d. preserves glycogen very well

79. Mercuric chloride pigment may be removed from tissue by:

   a. treating sections with an iodine-sodium thiosulfate sequence
   b. using a limonene clearing agent on the tissue processor
   c. rinsing sections with 50% to 70% alcohol
   d. washing sections with running water

80. To prevent the formation of formalin pigment in tissues, formalin should be:

   a. heated
   b. cooled
   c. buffered
   d. acidified

81. Which of the following fixatives should be used for specimens that are to be mailed?

   a. 10% neutral buffered formalin
   b. Bouin solution
   c. Helly solution
   d. Zenker solution

82. A biopsy that was placed in water by mistake is submitted to the laboratory. This mistake most likely will cause:

   a. mushy sections
   b. swollen and ruptured cells
   c. hardening of the tissue
   d. no appreciable changes

83. Sections of a breast carcinoma were fixed in a saline solution in the microwave oven. Microscopic examination of H&E-stained sections show marked pyknotic, overstained nuclei. The staining results were most likely caused by the:

   a. use of saline for fixation
   b. solution temperature exceeding 55°C
   c. use of plastic containers in the microwave
   d. presence of carcinoma in the breast tissue

84. An unknown pigment in a tissue section that can be bleached with a saturated alcoholic solution of picric acid is most likely:

   a. melanin pigment
   b. formalin pigment
   c. hemosiderin
   d. mercury pigment

85. The formaldehyde in Helly solution:

   a. causes reduction of some chemicals in the solution
   b. coagulates and denatures tissue proteins
   c. prevents turbidity and precipitate formation
   d. eliminates the need for post-fixation washing

86. Formaldehyde solutions for routine use are most commonly buffered by:

   a. monobasic and dibasic phosphates
   b. sodium acetate and acetic acid
   c. s-collidine and hydrochloric acid
   d. sodium barbitol and sodium hydroxide

87. If asked to cut cryostat sections of tissue fixed in Zenker solution, the histotechnologist should:

   a. section the tissue as is
   b. explain that frozen sections containing mercuric chloride cannot be made
   c. treat the tissue with iodine, hypo, and water before freezing
   d. use a solution of 30% sucrose to infiltrate the tissue before freezing

88. One characteristic of Zamboni fixative is that it:

   a. does not stabilize cellular proteins
   b. is recommended for electron microscopy
   c. is easily destroyed by tissue fluids
   d. must be followed by osmium tetroxide

89. The best fixative for blood smears is:

    a. Bouin solution
    b. Carnoy solution
    c. B-5 solution
    d. methanol

90. When used as a secondary fixative, osmium tetroxide should be:

    a. used after lead citrate
    b. heated prior to use
    c. combined with alcohol
    d. used under a chemical hood

91. Which of the following fixatives is recommended for use in lipid histochemistry?

    a. Zenker solution
    b. acetone
    c. formalin-saline
    d. calcium-formalin

92. In the Cajal method for demonstrating astrocytes, sections of brain should be fixed in formalin that contains:

    a. sodium acetate
    b. ammonium bromide
    c. mercuric chloride
    d. calcium chloride

93. Hollande solution is a modification of which of the following fixatives?

    a. Helly solution
    b. Orth solution
    c. Carnoy solution
    d. Bouin solution

94. Tissue fixed in which of the following solutions must be post-treated for mercuric chloride pigment?

    a. B-5
    b. Zamboni
    c. Carnoy
    d. Orth

95. Acetone is recommended for the primary fixation of:

    a. prostate tissue for immunohistochemistry
    b. kidney tissue for fluorescent antibody techniques
    c. muscle tissue for enzyme histochemistry
    d. brain tissue for the diagnosis of rabies

96. Fresh, unfixed tissue can be stored safely for a short time by:

   a. keeping it in a freezer
   b. wrapping it in saline-moistened gauze and refrigerating it
   c. placing it in physiological saline at room temperature
   d. leaving it in a dry specimen container on the counter with a note to
      the histologist

97. Zenker solution contains:

   a. mercuric chloride, potassium dichromate, and formaldehyde
   b. mercuric chloride, chromic acid, and formaldehyde
   c. mercuric chloride, potassium dichromate, and acetic acid
   d. potassium dichromate, formaldehyde, and acetic acid

98. One characteristic of Bouin solution is that it:

   a. penetrates poorly
   b. destroys delicate structures
   c. mordants connective tissue stains
   d. preserves erythrocytes

99. The fixation of tissue by physical methods can be demonstrated by the use of:

   a. microincineration
   b. microwaves
   c. frozen sections
   d. alcohol

100. Fixation in Carnoy solution will result in:

   a. swelling of the tissue
   b. preservation of most cytoplasmic structures
   c. superior staining of amyloid with Congo red
   d. good preservation of red blood cells

101. The recommended fixative for tissue suspected of containing spirochetes is:

   a. 10% neutral buffered formalin
   b. Bouin solution
   c. Zenker solution
   d. Helly solution

102. Which of the following is frequently added to formalin solutions to help preserve immunoreactivity?

   a. glycerin
   b. sodium acetate
   c. zinc salts
   d. chromates

103. Which of the following fixatives is recommended for both the Heidenhain and Mallory aniline blue stains?

   a. Orth fluid
   b. neutral buffered formalin
   c. Zenker fluid
   d. absolute ethanol

104. A fixative used for the preservation of some enzymes is:

   a. Bouin solution
   b. B-5 solution
   c. acetone
   d. isopropanol

105. A common reason for adding acetic acid to fixatives is to:

   a. coagulate proteins
   b. reduce shrinkage
   c. preserve carbohydrates
   d. change the pH

106. Formaldehyde acts as a fixative by:

   a. uncovering acid groups
   b. coagulating proteins
   c. cross-linking proteins
   d. rupturing peptide linkages

107. When it is known prior to fixation that a distinction must be made between collagen and muscle, the preferred fixative is:

   a. neutral buffered formalin
   b. Orth fluid
   c. absolute alcohol
   d. Bouin fluid

108. For optimum staining results, Bouin or Zenker fixation is recommended for:

   a. the Wilder reticulum technique
   b. most trichrome stains
   c. the Weigert elastic tissue stain
   d. any silver stain

109. In Bouin fixative, the shrinking effect produced by one component is balanced by the swelling effect of:

   a. formalin
   b. acetic acid
   c. osmium tetroxide
   d. potassium dichromate

110. 10% formalin is equivalent to what percent paraformaldehyde?

    a. 40
    b. 10
    c. 4
    d. 1

111. The use of formalin as a fixative in the microwave oven:

    a. is a possible explosive hazard
    b. produces toxic vapors
    c. degrades plastic cassettes
    d. corrodes fixed tissues

112. Which of the following renders fat insoluble for subsequent processing?

    a. picric acid
    b. osmium tetroxide
    c. chloroform
    d. formaldehyde

113. The presence of acetic acid in fixatives produces:

    a. cell shrinkage
    b. red cell destruction
    c. protein coagulation
    d. lipid preservation

114. Microscopic review of a formalin-fixed tissue section demonstrates a fine, brown-black artifactual pigment. This artifact most likely could have been prevented by:

    a. placing the tissue in formalin immediately after removal
    b. preparing the solution just before use
    c. washing the tissue after fixation
    d. making the solution neutral

115. When osmium tetroxide is used as a fixative, it:

    a. must be used after a primary fixative
    b. should be used in a hood
    c. should be made hypotonic to tissue
    d. must be made basic

116. Which of the following fixative components produces shrinkage and penetrates poorly:

    a. glacial acetic acid
    b. mercuric chloride
    c. potassium dichromate
    d. ethanol

117. The component in Bouin solution that causes tissue shrinkage is:

   a. picric acid
   b. acetic acid
   c. mercuric chloride
   d. potassium dichromate

118. Which of the following fixatives should be selected when it is desirable to preserve erythrocytes in tissue?

   a. Zenker
   b. Bouin
   c. Carnoy
   d. B-5

119. A tissue section reveals a dark brown microcrystalline pigment which is birefringent. To remove this pigment, the section should be treated with an alcoholic solution saturated with:

   a. sodium thiosulfate
   b. oxalic acid
   c. picric acid
   d. hydrochloric acid

120. Shrinkage and distortion of tissue is greatest following fixation in:

   a. Zenker fluid
   b. Bouin fluid
   c. absolute alcohol
   d. Helly fluid

121. Tissue to be stained by the Warthin-Starry technique should be fixed in:

   a. Zenker fluid
   b. saturated mercuric chloride
   c. formalin
   d. osmium tetroxide

122. Alcohol, rather than water, is used as the solvent in some fixatives because alcohol:

   a. helps precipitate proteins
   b. decreases tissue shrinkage
   c. increases lipid preservation
   d. eliminates the need for dehydration

123. When preparing Helly solution, formalin should be added:

   a. when other ingredients are combined
   b. before adding mercuric chloride
   c. when ready to use
   d. 24 hours before use

124. When fat is to be preserved, the fixative of choice is:

    a. formalin
    b. Zenker solution
    c. Carnoy solution
    d. Bouin solution

125. Picric acid was used alone as a fixative for a section of liver. The tissue most likely will show:

    a. extreme swelling
    b. excessive hardening
    c. an increased uptake of eosin
    d. hydrolyzed nucleic acids

126. The primary purpose of fixation is the:

    a. preservation of carbohydrates
    b. coagulation of lipids
    c. removal of tissue fluids
    d. stabilization of proteins

127. Bouin solution lyses erythrocytes because of it contains:

    a. formalin
    b. picric acid
    c. acetic acid
    d. alcohol

The following items (*) have been identified as more appropriate for entry-level histotechnologists.

* 128. Microscopic examination of a PAS-stained section reveals marked nonspecific staining. This could be caused by fixation in:

    a. Bouin solution
    b. Gendre solution
    c. 10% neutral buffered formalin
    d. glutaraldehyde solution

* 129. The pathologist is sure that urate crystals were present in a tissue biopsy and should therefore be present in the H&E-stained section, but polarization of the tissue is negative. This could possibly result from the:

    a. application of the wrong stain for demonstration
    b. poor clearing and infiltration of the biopsy
    c. fact that urate crystals are not birefringent
    d. use of a water-based fixative

* 130. Formaldehyde reacts primarily with which of the following protein groups?

    a. COOH
    b. C=O
    c. NH_2
    d. N=N

* 131. During embedding, a white deposit is noted on several of tissues. The tissues had been fixed in zinc-formalin, transferred to phosphate-buffered formalin, dehydrated with 65%, 95%, and absolute alcohols, and cleared with xylene. One possible explanation of the white deposit could be that the tissue was:

    a. left in the zinc-formalin too long
    b. fixed in incompatible fixatives
    c. improperly washed between formalin solutions
    d. not dehydrated appropriately for the method of fixation

* 132. Electron micrographs of a tissue section reveal electron-lucent membranes. This most likely indicates that:

    a. fixation was done in Bouin solution
    b. the osmolality of the fixative was incorrect
    c. the specimen was not post-fixed in osmium tetroxide
    d. sections were stained with uranyl acetate

* 133. Michel medium is:

    a. used for transporting unfixed tissue
    b. indicated for long-term storage of fixed tissue
    c. a fixative with limited use
    d. an antigen retrieval solution

* 134. Microscopic evaluation of H&E-stained sections from a surgically removed, formalin-fixed small bowel specimen show an absence of much of the epithelium in otherwise normal tissue. This could most likely be prevented in the future by:

    a. opening the specimen and adding fixative upon receipt
    b. avoiding the use of forceps during the dissection
    c. allowing the specimen to fix for 48 hours
    d. increasing the percentage of formalin in the solution

* 135. Recently a laboratory's primary fixative has been changed from neutral buffered formalin to an alcohol-based fixative promoted for antigen preservation. A marked difference in H&E staining is noted, with a marked increase in eosin uptake. This most likely results from the new fixative:

a. creating a different tissue isoelectric point
b. blocking protein precipitation
c. generating more negative charges
d. increasing cross-linking of the amino group

* 136. Microscopic evaluation of an H&E-stained section fixed in 10% neutral buffered formalin shows a complete absence of the surface epithelium and poor cellular detail in the lamina propria. This is most likely the result of:

a. autolysis
b. mechanical trauma
c. antemortem changes
d. prolonged fixation

* 137. When sucrose is used to treat tissue for enzyme histochemical studies:

a. cell membranes are mobilized
b. frozen sectioning is very difficult
c. the tissue must be removed after a brief period of treatment
d. the solution should contain 30% sucrose and 1% gum acacia

* 138. Kidney tissue has been submitted in Michel medium for immunofluorescence studies. Before the histotechnologist performs the required studies, the tissue should be:

a. washed in PBS containing 10% sucrose
b. frozen immediately upon receipt
c. placed in an aldehyde fixative
d. refrigerated

* 139. An isotonic solution for human tissue has an osmolality of approximately:

a. 500 milliosmols
b. 340 milliosmols
c. 260 milliosmols
d. 150 milliosmols

* 140. Marked distortion of architecture and predominantly pyknotic nuclei are noted on H&E-stained sections of kidney tissue. The tissue was fixed in the microwave in a saline solution. This problem could most likely have been prevented by:

a. changing the processing schedule
b. using another fixative solution
c. carefully controlling the temperature
d. using longer fixation times

* 141. Paraffin blocks containing tissue fixed in Bouin solution are retrieved from storage after several years. New sections are cut and stained with H&E, and no nuclear staining is present, although the nuclei of the original slides were well-stained. To prevent this from happening in the future on tissue to be stored, one must:

a. neutralize the picric acid before processing
b. be sure that the pH of the Bouin solution is at neutrality
c. make certain that the formalin does not contain formic acid
d. store the blocks in a facility with a maximum temperature of 20°C

* 142. Microscopic examination of an H&E-stained section fixed in formalin shows nuclear bubbling. This could most likely be avoided in the future by:

a. extending the length of fixation
b. fixing at refrigerator temperatures
c. changing the pH of the fixative
d. decreasing the osmolality of the fixative

* 143. During the examination of an electron microscopy print, it is noted that leaching of cellular material has occurred and that the cytomembrane appears to be "bubbling". This problem is most likely caused by fixing the tissue in osmium tetroxide for:

a. 1 minute
b. 30 minutes
c. 1 hour
d. overnight

* 144. Which of the following fixatives is stable at room temperature?

a. Karnovsky paraformaldehyde-glutaraldehyde
b. 2% to 3% glutaraldehyde
c. Zamboni PAF
d. 1% buffered osmium tetroxide

* 145. The paraformaldehyde in Karnovsky paraformaldehyde-glutaraldehyde solution must be heated to 60°C prior to adding the 1 M NaOH in order to:

a. dissociate the paraformaldehyde
b. purify the glutaraldehyde
c. polymerize the glutaraldehyde
d. eliminate the gasses present

* 146. Prior to processing, tissue fixed in glutaraldehyde for electron microscopy should be:

a. post-fixed in formaldehyde
b. rinsed with gum sucrose solution
c. post-fixed in osmium tetroxide solution
d. rinsed with an alcohol buffer solution

* 147. Poor fixation of electron microscopy specimens will be indicated by the appearance of:

    a. evenly dispersed ground substance
    b. stabilized cytoplasmic proteins
    c. displaced mitochondrial membranes
    d. unaltered nuclear and cytoplasmic membranes

* 148. Formalin pigment may be removed from microscopic sections by treating them with:

    a. Lugol's iodine and sodium thiosulfate
    b. potassium permanganate
    c. dilute acetic acid
    d. potassium hydroxide in 80% alcohol

* 149. Fixatives producing covalent bonding that tends to mask antigenic sites and hamper immunohisto-chemical localization of antigens contain:

    a. mercury
    b. phosphates
    c. aldehydes
    d. alcohol

* 150. For which of the following techniques are frozen sections of fixed tissue preferred?

    a. autoradiography of steroid hormones
    b. enzyme histochemistry of muscle biopsies
    c. fat stains of liver
    d. fluorescent antibody techniques

* 151. In immuno-electron microscopy (IEM), a fixative other than osmium tetroxide is used because osmium would:

    a. blacken the tissue
    b. block entrance of the gold label
    c. destroy the antigenicity of the sample
    d. decrease membrane preservation

* 152. The difference between Orth and Helly solutions is that ONLY Helly contains:

    a. formaldehyde
    b. potassium dichromate
    c. mercuric chloride
    d. acetic acid

* 153. A small biopsy is submitted with a request for "stat" acid-fast and fungus stains. The tissue should be fixed in:

    a. Zenker solution
    b. Carnoy fluid
    c. B-5 fluid
    d. buffered formalin

* 154. A microwave oven can be used for fixation because it:

   a. causes cross-linking of proteins
   b. induces physical fixation
   c. increases tissue basophilia
   d. inactivates enzymes with beta radiation

* 155. Unstained slides from B-5–fixed tissue should be treated with which of the following before staining?

   a. lithium carbonate
   b. potassium iodide
   c. sodium bisulfite
   d. iodine

* 156. Microscopic evaluation of a tissue section reveals a brown pigment lying on top of the tissue. Adjacent sections are treated with:
   1. iodine and sodium thiosulfate
   2. potassium ferrocyanide and hydrochloric acid
   3. saturated alcoholic solution of picric acid

   All sections still show the brown pigment. This pigment could have resulted from improper washing following fixation in:

   a. Zenker fluid
   b. formalin
   c. B-5 fluid
   d. Bouin fluid

* 157. A possible rhabdomyosarcoma is brought to the laboratory for appropriate fixation. For the non-immunohistochemical stains needed to confirm this tumor, at least one section should be fixed in:

   a. Orth fluid
   b. Bouin fluid
   c. Zenker fluid
   d. buffered formalin

* 158. Tissue fixed in osmium tetroxide must be:

   a. washed with running water
   b. cut very thin for fixation
   c. fixed overnight before processing
   d. processed on a short cycle

* 159. When osmium tetroxide is used on a kidney biopsy for ultrastructural studies, the time of fixation:

   a. is not critical
   b. should be one hour or less
   c. is prolonged because of tissue density
   d. depends on the fixative concentration

* 160. Helly fixative prepared 3 weeks previously is now discolored and turbid. The most likely reason for this is:

   a. the presence of acetic acid in the fixative
   b. improper solution buffering
   c. the premature addition of formaldehyde
   d. chemical oxidation

*161. A stained microscopic section shows marked lysis of erythrocytes, amorphous brown pigment lying on top of the section, and pale nuclear staining. These results indicate improper treatment after fixation in:

   a. formalin
   b. Helly fluid
   c. Zenker fluid
   d. Orth fluid

* 162. A small amount of white precipitate is noticed in the bottom of the laboratory's stock 37% to 40% formaldehyde container. The most appropriate action is to:

   a. discard the solution
   b. disregard the precipitate
   c. acidify the solution slightly
   d. add methanol to the solution

* 163. Acetone can be used to fix tissue for the demonstration of:

   a. myelin sheaths
   b. phospholipids
   c. oxidoreductases
   d. cell surface antigens

* 164. A tissue block of unfixed hemorrhagic spleen is fixed for 24 hours in formalin that was prepared 6 months previously. Subsequent H&E-stained sections show a granular black pigment on the surface of the tissue. This problem can most likely be prevented in the future by:

   a. washing the tissue prior to fixation
   b. ensuring that the formalin contains buffering reagents
   c. using an iodine solution on the processor
   d. using only freshly prepared solutions

* 165. Zenker fixation is critical for a nonimmunohistochemical special stain used in the diagnosis of which of the following tumors?

   a. liposarcoma
   b. fibrosarcoma
   c. neurosarcoma
   d. rhabdomyosarcoma

* 166. Tissue is received in Zenker fixative. After 72 hours of fixation, it is washed in running water for 12 hours, then routinely processed and stained with H&E. The nuclei appear very poorly stained. This problem can be corrected in the future by:

a. increasing the blueing time during staining
b. extending the washing time before processing
c. decreasing the fixation time
d. minimizing the slide drying time

* 167. A gouty tophus is seen in a fresh tissue specimen. The ideal fixative for the crystals which may be occurring with this condition is:

a. buffered formalin
b. Bouin fluid
c. absolute alcohol
d. Orth fluid

* 168. To ensure adequate fixation, a colon polyp measuring approximately 2 × 2 × 3 cm should be placed in, at the minimum, what volume of fixative?

a. 2.4 mL
b. 24 mL
c. 240 mL
d. 2400 mL

* 169. A characteristic of acetone fixation is that:

a. glycogen is removed from tissues
b. enzymes are removed from tissues
c. the tissues are overhardened
d. antigen-antibody reactions are destroyed

* 170. A wet tissue sample has been requested for electron microscopy. All available tissue has been fixed in Bouin solution, washed, and stored in 70% alcohol. Electron microscopy on the tissue would show:

a. good fixation of nucleoproteins
b. well-preserved organelles
c. some shrinkage of the nucleolus
d. inadequately preserved ultrastructures

* 171. A surgical specimen is obtained from a patient with a diagnosis of probable metastatic malignant melanoma. The choice of fixatives should be compatible with the use of which of the following special stains or diagnostic procedures?

a. colloidal iron
b. immunohistochemistry
c. immunofluorescence
d. digestion procedures

* 172. A section of tendon sheath has been fixed in 10% neutral buffered formalin for 24 hours, routinely processed, and embedded in paraffin. The demonstration of urate crystals on sections from this block:

    a. should be performed after post-fixation
    b. will be best with a fluorescence technique
    c. must be performed on air-dried sections
    d. will not be possible due to improper fixation

* 173. When Helly fluid has been used as a fixative, it is necessary to remove which of the following from the sample?

    a. mercury crystals
    b. picric acid
    c. formalin pigment
    d. iron pigment

* 174. A section of healthy adrenal gland to be used as a control for chromaffin granules is fixed in osmic acid for 8 hours. When examined microscopically, no granules are demonstrated. This problem can be resolved in the future by:

    a. washing the tissue before staining
    b. selecting another tissue for the control
    c. using another fixative
    d. increasing the fixation time

* 175. An aqueous fixative MUST be chosen for sections that require:

    a. the preservation of lipids
    b. rapid sample fixation
    c. maximum hardening
    d. preservation of amyloid

* 176. One of the functions of fixation is to:

    a. form insoluble tissue salts
    b. inhibit autolytic enzymes
    c. adjust the nuclear/cytoplasmic ratio
    d. maintain a neutral pH

* 177. Pap smears that have been fixed with a spray fixative are submirred to the laboratory. The smears are stained without an other treatment. The most likely result will be

    a. excellent cytological detail
    b. the loss of cells from the slide
    c. cells showing air-drying artifact
    d. nuclei that appear foggy and lack detail

* 178. Paraffin blocks of Bouin-fixed tissue have been stored for 2 years. Results of current tests show very poor H&E staining and some structural deterioration. However, the original sections from the blocks show excellent preservation and staining. The changes are most likely due to:

a. excessive heat during embedding
b. residual picric acid in the block
c. freezing of blocks during storage
d. physical changes in the paraffin

Fixation Answer Key

The following items have been identified as appropriate for both entry level histologic technicians and histotechnologists.

1. a	33. a	65. d	97. c
2. d	34. b	66. a	98. c
3. a	35. c	67. d	99. b
4. b	36. d	68. b	100. c
5. b	37. b	69. d	101. a
6. d	38. d	70. c	102. c
7. c	39. b	71. d	103. c
8. a	40. b	72. b	104. c
9. a	41. b	73. a	105. b
10. c	42. c	74. b	106. c
11. b	43. b	75. b	107. d
12. d	44. c	76. c	108. b
13. a	45. d	77. c	109. b
14. a	46. d	78. d	110. c
15. c	47. c	79. a	111. b
16. a	48. b	80. c	112. b
17. a	49. d	81. a	113. b
18. d	50. a	82. b	114. d
19. b	51. b	83. b	115. b
20. c	52. d	84. b	116. b
21. d	53. d	85. a	117. a
22. a	54. d	86. a	118. d
23. a	55. a	87. c	119. c
24. c	56. c	88. b	120. c
25. d	57. d	89. d	121. c
26. c	58. d	90. d	122. a
27. d	59. b	91. d	123. c
28. c	60. b	92. b	124. a
29. a	61. c	93. d	125. d
30. a	62. b	94. a	126. d
31. d	63. a	95. d	127. c
32. b	64. a	96. b	

The following items (*) have been identified as more appropriate for the entry level histotechnologists.

* 128. d	* 141. a	* 154. b	* 167. c
* 129. d	* 142. a	* 155. d	* 168. c
* 130. c	* 143. d	* 156. a	* 169. c
* 131. c	* 144. c	* 157. c	* 170. d
* 132. c	* 145. a	* 158. b	* 171. b
* 133. a	* 146. c	* 159. b	* 172. d
* 134. a	* 147. c	* 160. c	* 173. a
* 135. a	* 148. d	* 161. c	* 174. c
* 136. a	* 149. c	* 162. b	* 175. a
* 137. d	* 150. c	* 163. d	* 176. b
* 138. a	* 151. c	* 164. b	* 177. d
* 139. b	* 152. c	* 165. d	* 178. b
* 140. c	* 153. d	* 166. c	

Chapter 10

Laboratory Operations

The following items have been identified as appropriate for both entry-level histologic technicians and histotechnologists.

1. Which of the following protective equipment must be worn (by law) when one is handling formaldehyde?

   a. impervious apron
   b. lab coat
   c. scrub suit
   d. white uniform

2. The short-term exposure limit (STEL) for formaldehyde set by the Formaldehyde Standard is:

   a. 0.5 ppm
   b. 0.75 ppm
   c. 1.0 ppm
   d. 2.0 ppm

3. Which of the following may be disposed of in the sanitary sewer system according to Environmental Protection Agency (EPA) and Centers for Disease Control (CDC) guidelines?

   a. absolute alcohol
   b. silver salts
   c. pulverized tissue
   d. blood

4. 500 mL of a 0.55% solution of potassium metabisulfite must be prepared. How many grams of potassium metabisulfite should be used?

   a. 1.10
   b. 2.75
   c. 5.50
   d. 11.0

5. Which of the following hazard classifications is of primary concern with picric acid?

a. mechanical
b. biological
c. chemical
d. fire/explosion

6. The Formaldehyde Standard sets the time-weighted average (TWA) for formaldehyde at:

a. 0.5 ppm
b. 0.75 ppm
c. 1.0 ppm
d. 2.0 ppm

7. A temperature of 4°C is commonly associated with the laboratory:

a. flotation bath
b. incubator
c. refrigerator
d. freezer

8. Potassium dichromate falls into which of the following hazard classifications?

a. mechanical
b. biological
c. chemical
d. fire/explosion

9. Which of the following pHs is considered basic?

a. 6.0
b. 6.5
c. 7.0
d. 7.5

10. A microscope with 2 eyepieces is:

a. monocular
b. binocular
c. achromatic
d. parfocal

11. When used in a National Fire Protection Association (NFPA) diamond, which of the following numbers is indicative of the most severe hazard?

a. 1
b. 2
c. 3
d. 4

12. Flammability hazards are indicated in which section of the NFPA diamond?

    a. blue
    b. red
    c. yellow
    d. white

13. According to the Environmental Protection Agency, it is illegal to dispose of concentrated acetic acid in the sanitary sewer system because it is classified as:

    a. carcinogenic
    b. corrosive
    c. oxidizing
    d. non-biodegradable

14. How many mL of water should be added to 80 mL of concentrated formaldehyde to obtain a solution of 10% formalin?

    a. 360
    b. 720
    c. 800
    d. 920

15. During microscopic examination, if the section remains in focus when changing objectives, the objectives are:

    a. binocular
    b. achromatic
    c. apochromatic
    d. parfocal

16. Paraffin sections of brain are cut at 15 micrometers. This is equivalent to how many millimeters?

    a. 1.5
    b. 0.15
    c. 0.015
    d. 0.0015

17. A 0.5% solution of light green is needed. The bottle contains only 4.25 grams of dye powder. How many mL of solution can be prepared if all of the dye is used?

    a. 212
    b. 425
    c. 850
    d. 1700

18. The handling of biohazards is governed by the:

   a. Blood-borne Pathogen Standard
   b. Formaldehyde Standard
   c. Laboratory Standard
   d. Respiratory Protection Standard

19. A solution is prepared that contains 5 g of NaCl in 200 mL of water. This is equivalent to which of the following percent solutions?

   a. 0.4
   b. 1.0
   c. 2.5
   d. 5.0

20. A dye solution that is applied after the primary stain has acted is called a(n):

   a. accentuator
   b. counterstain
   c. mordant
   d. differentiator

21. Hydrochloric acid may be disposed of in the sink, provided it is:

   a. diluted to 24%
   b. less than a 2N solution
   c. neutralized to a pH between 3 and 11
   d. not a concentrated solution

22. If a reagent is biodegradable, the disposal is always:

   a. in the sanitary sewer system
   b. as hazardous waste
   c. determined by water solubility
   d. by incineration

23. To obtain a total magnification of 1000 with an ocular of 10× magnification, the objective must have a magnification of:

   a. 10×
   b. 100×
   c. 450×
   d. 1000×

24. Fires involving wood and paper are considered:

    a. Class A fires
    b. Class B fires
    c. Class C fires
    d. Class D fires

25. During microscopic review of H&E-stained sections, it is noted that there is insufficient light on the slide. The best way to correct this is by:

    a. changing to a higher objective
    b. increasing the numerical aperture
    c. lowering the substage condenser
    d. opening the iris diaphragm

26. Organic solvents should be disposed of by:

    a. pouring them down a sink and flushing with plenty of water
    b. collecting them in waste containers for future disposal or distillation
    c. pouring them into a deep pit in the ground
    d. collecting them in old bottles and storing in a vacant building

27. 500 mL of 3% alcian blue in 1% acetic acid contains:

    a. 1 g alcian blue, 3 mL acetic acid, and 497 mL water
    b. 3 g alcian blue, 1 mL acetic acid, and 499 mL water
    c. 15 g alcian blue, 5 mL acetic acid, and 495 mL water
    d. 15 g alcian blue, 1 mL acetic acid, and 499 mL water

28. Another way of expressing 350 mg is as:

    a. 3.50 g
    b. 0.35 g
    c. 0.035 g
    d. 0.0035 g

29. Following staining with a solution prepared from a new bottle of eosin dye powder, the color results are not the same as those obtained with the previously used eosin dye powder. The best course of action is to:

    a. discard the new dye and reorder
    b. use an eosin substitute
    c. try another formula for the new eosin
    d. determine whether both dyes have the same dye content

30. Components of living tissue do not require staining if they are to be examined by:

    a. fluorescent microscopy
    b. light microscopy
    c. phase contrast microscopy
    d. transmission electron microscopy

31. An acidic or basic substance added to a solution to prevent a change in pH is called a(n):

    a. differentiator
    b. oxidizer
    c. catalyst
    d. buffer

32. The "high-dry" objective usually has a magnification of:

    a. 4×
    b. 10×
    c. 20×
    d. 45×

33. A section 5 micrometers thick would be equivalent to how many millimeters in thickness?

    a. 0.0005
    b. 0.005
    c. 0.05
    d. 0.5

34. Individual virus particles cannot be seen by light microscopy, but can be visualized by:

    a. phase microscopy
    b. polarizing microscopy
    c. electron microscopy
    d. fluorescence microscopy

35. How much 95% alcohol must be used to prepare 1000 mL of 70% alcohol?

    a. 271 mL
    b. 316 mL
    c. 714 mL
    d. 737 mL

36. Nontoxic, basic stains that are suspended in sterile water and injected into living animals are referred to as:

    a. vital
    b. in vitro
    c. amphoteric
    d. anionic

37. To prepare 50 mL of 2% ferric chloride from a 10% solution, how many mL of the 10% solution will be required?

    a. 5
    b. 10
    c. 20
    d. 25

38. Doubly refractile particles are also called:

    a. isotropic
    b. fluorescent
    c. birefringent
    d. reflective

39. Tissue can be fixed in the microwave oven because it causes:

    a. rapid molecular movement
    b. reaction between protein molecules
    c. ionizing radiation
    d. rupture of hydrogen bonds

40. How many mL of water should be added to 100 mL of a 20% solution of silver nitrate to obtain a 10% solution?

    a. 20
    b. 50
    c. 100
    d. 200

41. To prepare 500 mL of 0.55% potassium metabisulfite solution, how many grams of potassium metabisulfite would be required?

    a. 1.10
    b. 2.75
    c. 5.50
    d. 11.0

42. A reagent labeled with a NFPA diamond has a 4 in the blue quadrant. This means that:

    a. there is no hazard
    b. there is a slight hazard
    c. the material may be harmful if inhaled or absorbed
    d. the hazard is extreme and exposure could result in death

43. Before adjusting the pH of the Warthin-Starry staining solution, the pH meter should be calibrated with a buffer solution of pH:

   a. 4.0
   b. 6.0
   c. 7.0
   d. 10.0

44. One cubic centimeter is equal to:

   a. 0.01 liter
   b. 0.1 liter
   c. 1 milliliter
   d. 10 milliliters

45. Some striated muscle cells are as much as 400 millimeters in length. This is equivalent to how many centimeters?

   a. 0.04
   b. 0.4
   c. 4.0
   d. 40

46. The ability of a microscope objective to separate small detail is the:

   a. numerical aperture
   b. depth of focus
   c. virtual image
   d. resolving power

47. A fire involving hydrocarbon reagents is classified as a:

   a. Class A fire
   b. Class B fire
   c. Class C fire
   d. Class D fire

48. Which of the following reactions describes the process of reducing silver to its visible metallic state without the aid of extraneous agents?

   a. argentaffin
   b. decidual
   c. argyrophilic
   d. luteinizing

49. The primary purpose of the Biological Stain Commission is to certify that dye:

    a. contents are correct
    b. meets OSHA requirements
    c. meets all qualities required by the Commission
    d. is produced by a licensed company

50. A temperature of 37°C is most commonly associated with:

    a. the flotation bath
    b. the laboratory incubator
    c. paraffin infiltration
    d. room temperature

51. A gradual increase in staining time, with worsening overstaining, is noted when using a microwave oven equipped with a temperature probe. The first step in correcting this problem would be to:

    a. purchase a new temperature probe
    b. have the microwave oven repaired
    c. clean the temperature probe
    d. reposition the staining container

52. How many mL of 29% ferric chloride stock solution should be used when preparing 50 mL of 2% ferric chloride?

    a. 1.16
    b. 3.45
    c. 6.90
    d. 7.25

53. Which of the following is the formula for calculating a percent (w/v) solution?

    a. (grams of solute × 100)/(volume of solvent)
    b. (grams of solute) × (volume of solvent) × (100)
    c. (volume of solvent × 100)/(grams of solute)
    d. (grams of solute) × (volume of solvent)/(100)

54. How many mL of 10% sodium hydroxide are required to prepare 200 mL of a 4% solution?

    a. 8
    b. 20
    c. 40
    d. 80

55. Solvent recovery systems are able to separate contaminants from solvents because the contaminants:

    a. are acids and the solvents are bases
    b. differ in boiling points from the solvents
    c. differ in solubility from the solvents
    d. are larger molecules than the solvents

56. During a microwave Grocott staining procedure, the methenamine-silver reagent boils. In response to this, one should:

   a. not be concerned; this is an expected event
   b. decrease the heating time of the reagent
   c. use a larger container for the reagent
   d. switch to a different staining procedure

57. When fractional distillation solvent recovery systems are used, xylene:

   a. can be recycled only a limited number of times
   b. will be of higher purity recycled than when original
   c. cannot be completely separated from alcohol
   d. that is recovered should not be used for clearing

58. What volume of a stock solution of 25% NaCl would be required to prepare 250 mL of a 5% solution?

   a. 5 mL
   b. 12.5 mL
   c. 25 mL
   d. 50 mL

59. To help prevent back strain, the hips should form an angle of _____ degrees between trunk and thighs when a technician is seated at the microtome.

   a. 30° to 60°
   b. 60° to 90°
   c. 90° to 120°
   d. 120° to 150°

60. Polarizing microscopes use a polarizer and a(n):

   a. barrier filter
   b. diffuser
   c. analyzer
   d. refractometer

61. A researcher asks that sections of his tissue be cut at 70 micrometers. This is equivalent to how many millimeters in thickness?

   a. 0.0007
   b. 0.007
   c. 0.07
   d. 0.7

62. A solution contains 20 g of solute dissolved in 0.5 L of water. What is the percentage of this solution?

   a. 2%
   b. 4%
   c. 10%
   d. 20%

63. How many milliliters of a 3% solution can be made if 6 grams of solute are used?

   a. 100 mL
   b. 200 mL
   c. 400 mL
   d. 600 mL

64. When a solution containing hydrochloric acid is to be discarded in the sink, it should be:

   a. neutralized to pH 7.0
   b. between pH 3 and pH 11
   c. diluted to less than 24%
   d. followed by an alkaline solution

65. A small electrical fire occurs in the laboratory. Which of the following substances would be appropriate for use in extinguishing the fire?

   a. water
   b. soda acid
   c. carbon tetrachloride
   d. carbon dioxide

66. Microscopic review of slides stained for the presence of microorganisms requires the use of immersion oil. The purpose of the oil is to:

   a. enhance color contrast
   b. decrease the refractive index
   c. improve the resolution
   d. require less light intensity

67. Microwaves are produced by a(n):

   a. cathode ray tube
   b. magnetron
   c. electron gun
   d. halogen lamp

68. One micron is equal to:

   a. 0.001 meters
   b. 0.0001 meters
   c. 0.00001 meters
   d. 0.000001 meters

69. A chemical that should be used under a hood because of the possibility of extreme respiratory irritation is:

   a. picric acid
   b. diaminobenzidine
   c. hydrochloric acid
   d. chromic acid

70. When using the microwave oven at an intermediate power setting, the technician notices that the oven light dims intermittently, accompanied by variations in sound levels. The most appropriate course of action is to:

    a. have the power supply checked
    b. unplug the oven immediately
    c. check for microwave leaks
    d. do nothing, the equipment is functioning normally

71. How many grams of aniline blue should be used to prepare 750 mL of a 5% solution?

    a. 3.8
    b. 37.5
    c. 50.0
    d. 75.0

72. A stock solution of Harris hematoxylin is being prepared for use in the routine H&E procedure. In order to link the dye to the tissue, which of the following must be added to the solution?

    a. mercuric oxide
    b. aluminum ammonium sulfate
    c. ferric chloride
    d. acetic acid

73. An employee has been complains of tingling or numbness in the hands, an aching neck, and shoulder and wrist pain. Referral to the health clinic would most likely reveal the the employee most likely has:

    a. bursitis
    b. carpal tunnel syndrome
    c. chronic repetitive trauma
    d. range of motion inadequacy

74. To meet most inspection criteria, the laboratory is expected to prepare procedure manual to conform to the guidelines published by the:

    a. Centers for Disease Control (CDC)
    b. College of American Pathologists (CAP)
    c. Joint Commission on Accreditation of Healthcare Organizations (JCAHO)
    d. National Committee for Clinical Laboratory Standards (NCCLS)

75. The function of the condenser on the light microscope is to:

    a. concentrate light on the tissue specimen
    b. magnify and resolve the image
    c. regulate the intensity of light illuminating the specimen
    d. furnish strongly divergent light to the specimen

76. The possibility of repetitive motion injury (RMI) may be reduced by:

    a. using a rocking motion of the flywheel when cutting paraffin sections
    b. tightly gripping the forceps when embedding and coverslipping
    c. removing the lid of each cassette with the left thumb
    d. utilizing an automated coverslipping system

77. When an inorganic substance is dissolved in water, the usual result is:

    a. the Tyndall effect
    b. colloidal dispersion
    c. ionization
    d. electrolysis

The following items (*) have been identified as more appropriate for entry-level histotechnologists.

* 78. 100 mL of a 1% solution of Luxol fast blue is needed. The old, stock dye had a dye concentration of 80% and the new preparation has a dye concentration of 84%. To achieve the same consistency in staining as with the old dye, how many grams of the new dye are required?

    a. 0.95
    b. 1.0
    c. 1.05
    d. 1.4

* 79. An employee wears a lab coat while assisting in the gross dissection area. This employee is later seen in the cafeteria in the same lab coat, indicating that:

    a. the employee needs further training
    b. lab coats should not be used in the gross dissection area
    c. only street clothes should be worn to the cafeteria
    d. the employee is conforming with a perfectly acceptable practice

* 80. How many grams of solute are required to prepare 500 mL of a 0.2 N solution of $CaCl_2$ (atomic weights are Ca = 40.08, Cl = 35.45)?

    a. 2.22
    b. 5.55
    c. 11.1
    d. 22.2

* 81. 1 ml of a 1:50 dilution of antibody is needed. How many microliters of the primary antibody would be needed?

    a. 0.2
    b. 2.0
    c. 20.0
    d. 200.0

* 82. Which of the following solutions is considered hazardous and may NOT be disposed of in the sanitary sewer system?

    a. silver nitrate
    b. copper sulfate
    c. zinc sulfate
    d. ferric chloride

* 83. 500 mL of a 0.25 M solution of $CaCl_2$ (atomic weights are Ca = 40.08, Cl = 35.45) is needed. How many grams of $CaCl_2$ are required?

    a. 1.39
    b. 6.94
    c. 13.87
    d. 27.75

* 84. The cryostat used in the surgical suite has stopped cooling properly. To be in compliance with the Blood-borne Pathogen Standard, before having someone service the equipment, the cryostat should:

    a. be decontaminated
    b. be allowed to air dry
    b. be cleaned of debris
    d. have the microtome removed

* 85. How many grams of Na_2SO_4 (atomic weights are Na = 23, S = 32, O = 16) are required to prepare 500 mL of a 2 M solution?

    a. 35.5
    b. 71.0
    c. 142.0
    d. 284.0

* 87. 500 mL of a 0.2% solution of light green is needed. The old, stock dye had a dye concentration of 90% and the new preparation has a dye concentration of 85%. To achieve the same consistency in staining as with the old dye, how many grams of the new dye are required?

    a. 0.85
    b. 0.94
    c. 1.06
    d. 1.88

old = 90%

New = 85%

* 87. Which of the following reactions is represented by:

$$3 Ag^0 + AuCl_3 \longrightarrow Au^0 + 3 AgCl$$

a. production of ammoniacal silver solution
b. formaldehyde reduction of silver ions
c. toning of silver by gold chloride
d. removal of unreacted silver by sodium thiosulfate

* 88. A visible image is achieved in transmission electron microscopy when:

a. electrons passing through the specimen collide with a fluorescent-coated viewing screen
b. an electron-sensitive photographic emulsion is applied to the viewing screen
c. ultraviolet light is introduced to the viewing screen
d. electrons passing through the object split and emit light in the visible light range

* 89. 100 μL (microliters) equals:

a. 0.1 mL
b. 0.01 mL
c. 0.001 mL
d. 0.0001 mL

* 90. What is the normality of a solution containing 35.0 g of KOH (MW = 56) in sufficient water to make 500 mL of solution?

a. 0.7
b. 0.8
c. 1.25
d. 2.8

* 91. Plastic resins require more specialized handling techniques than waxes because resins:

a. may cause dermatitis
b. require manual embedding
c. are used at high temperatures
d. harden instantly

* 92. In electron microscopy, the electron beam is focused onto a specific specimen plane by varying the:
   a. strength of the electromagnetic fields
   b. output of the tungsten filaments
   c. length of the focal lenses
   d. position of the fluorescent screen

* 93. How many grams of NaOH (MW = 40) are required to prepare 500 mL of a 0.25 M solution?

   a. 5
   b. 10
   c. 12.5
   d. 20

* 94. The primary antibody must be diluted 1:100 for an immunohistochemical procedure. How many microliters of the primary antibody would be required to prepare a total volume of 2 mL?

   a. 2
   b. 10
   c. 20
   d. 100

* 95. 100 mL of 0.2 N KCl (MW = 74.55) contains how many grams of KCl?

   a. 0.75
   b. 1.49
   c. 7.46
   d. 14.9

* 96. Which of the following lenses is used in an electron microscope?

   a. glass
   b. mirrors
   c. tungsten filament
   d. electromagnetic coils

* 97. The use of chloroform in the histology laboratory requires safety precautions because it is:

   a. very reactive
   b. flammable
   c. a carcinogen
   d. corrosive

* 98. When compared with the light source in a standard light microscope, the electron microscope equivalent would be a(n):

   a. ultraviolet light
   b. halogen lamp
   c. electron beam
   d. roentgen rays

* 99. Substances that are recognized as foreign by the immune system are called:

    a. antibodies
    b. substrates
    c. antigens
    d. immunoglobulins

* 100. What is the normality of a solution which contains 280 grams of NaOH (MW = 40) in 2000 mL of solution?

    a. 3.5 N
    b. 5.5 N
    c. 7.0 N
    d. 8.0 N

* 101. A change in the pH of a solution from 7 to 6 indicates that the solution now contains:

    a. double the number of hydronium ions as before
    b. 5 times the number of hydronium ions as before
    c. 10 times the number of hydronium ions as before
    d. double the number of hydroxyl ions as before

* 102. How many grams of NaOH (MW = 40) are required to prepare a liter of 1 N NaOH?

    a. 13
    b. 20
    c. 40
    d. 80

* 103. An aqueous mounting medium was prepared 3 months previously and stored in a 4°C refrigerator. Mold is now observed in the medium. To prevent this in the future, when preparing the medium one should:

    a. be sure to add thymol
    b. filter the newly made solution
    c. increase the amount of glycerol
    d. boil the solution

* 104. Which of the following agencies provide fire safety standards that must be followed in the laboratory?

    a. ASCP and CAP
    b. FDA and HCFA
    c. OSHA and NFPA
    d. NSH and AMA

* 105. The terminology used to define the statistical average value is:

    a. mode
    b. median
    c. mean
    d. coefficient

* 106. A check of a known-positive control section from a Grocott procedure reveals the absence of stained organisms. This error may be avoided in the future by ensuring that:

    a. bacteria are present in the control section
    b. aldehyde groups are formed before impregnation
    c. chemical reducing agents are used
    d. the glassware is chemically cleaned

* 107. A solution of $Ca(OH)_2$ (molecular weight = 74) contains a 9.25 grams of the solute in 100 mL of solution. What is the normality of this solution?

    a. 2.5 N
    b. 3.7 N
    c. 7.4 N
    d. 9.2 N

* 108. After receipt of formaldehyde monitoring results, management must notify employees within how many days?

    a. 15
    b. 30
    c. 45
    d. 60

* 109. Given the following values:

    100
    120
    150
    140
    130

What is the mean?

    a. 100
    b. 128
    c. 130
    d. 640

* 110. The overtime budget for the laboratory is $38,773, but $50,419 has already been spent. What percent over budget does this represent?

   a. 33%
   b. 70%
   c. 77%
   d. 100%

* 111. A one normal solution is equivalent to:

   a. 1 mole of solute per kilogram of solvent
   b. 1 mole of solute per 100 mL of solution
   c. 1 gram-equivalent weight of solute per 1L of solution
   d. 2 moles of solute per 1L of solution

* 112. Which of the following is the formula for calculating the gram-equivalent weight of a chemical?

   a. MW × oxidation number
   b. MW/oxidation number
   c. MW + oxidation number
   d. MW − oxidation number

* 113. The proper microscope for examining tissue stained with thioflavin T is the:

   a. electron
   b. light
   c. polarizing
   d. fluorescence

* 114. 600 μL of antiserum are added to 2400 μL of diluent will give a final dilution of:

   a. 1:5
   b. 1:50
   c. 1:500
   d. 1:5000

* 115. How many grams of H_2SO_4 (MW = 98) are in 750 mL of 3N H_2SO_4?

   a. 36
   b. 72
   c. 110
   d. 146

* 116. What is the molarity of a solution that contains 18.7 g of KCl (MW = 74.5) in 500 mL of water?

   a. 0.25
   b. 0.5
   c. 0.75
   d. 1.25

* 117. A dangerous materials warning system chart developed by the NFPA is in use in the laboratory. A reagent is identified with a red background and the number three (3). This indicates a compound that:

a. will cause irritation if not treated
b. is unstable and may spontaneously explode
c. is flammable and will easily ignite
d. should be stored in an explosion proof cabinet

* 118. To maximize the resolving power of a light microscope, the substage condenser should be adjusted to sharply focus the image of the:

a. condenser front lens
b. lamp filament
c. specimen slide
d. field diaphragm

* 119. The number of hours used to calculate the annual salary of a full-time employee is:

a. 1920
b. 1950
c. 2080
d. 2800

* 120. While using a 10× objective to view an H&E-stained section, the section appears bright with well-stained nuclei. When the objective is changed to 40×, the section appears dark and detail is obscured. This problem most likely could be corrected by:

a. restaining the section and decreasing the hematoxylin
b. slightly opening the iris diaphragm
c. using the 90× objective
d. cleaning the ocular

* 121. Which of the following is the formula for calculating the molarity of a solution?

a. number of moles of solute per liter of solution
b. number of moles of solute × 100
c. 1 GEW of solute × 10
d. 1 GEW of solute per liter of solution

* 122. How many mL of 85% alcohol is required to make up 5000 mL of 60% alcohol?

a. 352.94
b. 2607.40
c. 3529.40
d. 3534.90

* 123. How many milliliters of 0.25 N NaOH are needed to make 100 mL of a 0.05 N solution of NaOH?

    a. 5
    b. 10
    c. 15
    d. 20

* 124. The best way to minimize the medical-legal and financial impact of losing computerized data through voltage variations is to:

    a. maintain a specimen logbook
    b. keep duplicate records
    c. perform frequent system backups
    d. install an electrical surge protector

* 125. The gross dissection area is being remodeled. Ventilation must be designed to ensure that the exposure to formaldehyde over an 8-hour period, or the time-weighted average (TWA), is no more than:

    a. 0.5 ppm
    b. 0.75 ppm
    c. 1.0 ppm
    d. 1.5 ppm

* 126. The middle value of a data set is statistically known as the:

    a. mean
    b. median
    c. mode
    d. standard deviation

* 127. The time-weighted average (TWA) of exposure to formaldehyde has been shown by monitoring to be 0.7 parts per million. According to OSHA regulations for the permissible exposure limit (PEL), the TWA must be:

    a. corrected within 15 days
    b. re-monitored within 15 days
    c. re-monitored within 6 months
    d. reported to the employee within 5 days

* 128. Tissue is submitted for cell membrane studies. The method of choice for these studies uses which of the following microscopes?

    a. electron
    b. phase
    c. polarizing
    d. light

129.* The microscopist is examining an FITC-stained section with a fluorescence microscope and thinks that there is some background autofluoresence. Of the following, which is most likely to autofluoresce?

a. muscle striations
b. urate crystals
c. talc or silica
d. elastic fibers

*130. The numerical aperture of the objective lens:

a. is unaffected by immersion media
b. defines the expected resolving power of the microscope
c. increases as the resolving power of the microscope decreases
d. is greater with a high dry objective than with an oil immersion objective

*131. CAP requires that approximately 90% of routine specimens requiring a frozen section have a turn-around-time (calculated from arrival in the grossing area to notification of the diagnosis measuring:

a. 15 minutes
b. 20 minutes
c. 25 minutes
d. 30 minutes

*132. While examining an H&E stained section of kidney, the microscopist encounters a problem with continual blurring through the left ocular. The blurring will most likely be eliminated by:

a. removing the left ocular and cleaning with xylene
b. removing the coverslip from the stained slide and replacing with a new clean coverslip focusing the microscope sharply to the right eye, then closing the right eye and adjusting
c. the left ocular until the image is sharp for the left eye.
d. assuming that the microscope is not parfocal and that nothing can be done to make the focus correct for both eyes

*133. Which of the following inquiries legally can be made regarding a job applicant's affiliations?

a. private organization affiliations
b. specific jobs, social organizations or experiences that relate the position the applicant is seeking
c. religious affiliations of the applicant, including any holidays observed
d. political affiliations

*134. The means by which an employee knows what is expected of him/her is known as the:

    a. work schedule
    b. procedure manual
    c. job description
    d. job analysis

*135. A histology tissue processor costs $42,000, has a life expectancy of 6 years and a guaranteed trade-in value of $8,000, and will handle 9000 specimens a year. Calculate its yearly depreciation allowance using straight-line depreciation.

    a $7750
    b. $5666
    c. $34,000
    d. $3777

*136. The Histology section of the laboratory had 12,652 labor hours for the year. How many FTE's were used by this section?

    a. 4.4
    b. 5.7
    c. 6.1
    d. 9.2

*137. Which of the following describes the process of establishing and declaring that a person has met the standards established by a professional organization?

    a. accreditation
    b. certification
    c. credentialing
    d. licensure

Laboratory Operations Answer Key

The following items have been identified as appropriate for both entry level histologic technicians and histotechnologists.

1. a	21. c	41. b	61. c
2. d	22. c	42. d	62. b
3. d	23. b	43. a	63. b
4. b	24. a	44. c	64. b
5. d	25. d	45. d	65. d
6. b	26. b	46. d	66. c
7. c	27. c	47. b	67. b
8. c	28. b	48. a	68. d
9. d	29. d	49. c	69. c
10. b	30. c	50. b	70. d
11. d	31. d	51. c	71. b
12. b	32. d	52. b	72. b
13. b	33. b	53. a	73. c
14. b	34. c	54. d	74. d
15. d	35. d	55. b	75. a
16. c	36. a	56. b	76. d
17. c	37. b	57. b	77. c
18. a	38. c	58. d	
19. c	39. a	59. b	
20. b	40. c	60. c	

The following items (*) have been identified as more appropriate for the entry level histotechnologists.

* 78. a	* 93. a	* 108. a	* 123. d
* 79. a	* 94. c	* 109. b	* 124. d
* 80. b	* 95. b	* 110. a	* 125. b
* 81. c	* 96. d	* 111. c	* 126. b
* 82. a	* 97. c	* 112. b	* 127. c
* 83. c	* 98. c	* 113. d	* 128. a
* 84. a	* 99. c	* 114. a	* 129. a
* 85. b	* 100. a	* 115. c	* 130. b
* 86. b b	* 101. c	* 116. b	* 131. b
* 87. c	* 102. c	* 117. c	* 132. c
* 88. a	* 103. a	* 118. d	* 133. b
* 89. a	* 104. c	* 119. c	* 134. c
* 90. c	* 105. c	* 120. b	* 135. b
* 91. a	* 106. b	* 121. a	* 136. c
* 92. a	* 107. a	* 122. c	* 137. b

Chapter 11

Microtomy

The following items have been identified as appropriate for both histologic technicians and histotechnologists.

1. Which of the following can be used to soften the exposed face of paraffin-embedded tissue that is too hard to section, such as uterine tissue?

   a. acid
   b. glycerine
   c. heat
   d. xylene

2. The supplier sent paraffin with a melting point of 50° to 52°C by mistake. When compared to paraffin with a melting point of 55°C, this paraffin will:

   a. provide better support for hard tissues
   b. yield thinner sections
   c. ribbon more easily
   d. require a warmer flotation bath

3. A different kind of paraffin is under consideration for use in the laboratory. An important fact to remember is that as the melting point of paraffin is increased, the paraffin:

   a. becomes harder
   b. provides less support
   c. ribbons more easily
   d. yields thicker sections

4. To obtain a section of small bowel showing mucosa, sub-mucosa, muscularis externa, and adventitia, the tissue must be embedded:

   a. on edge
   b. at an angle
   c. epithelial surface up
   d. mucosal surface down

5. Holes are noted in a frozen section of skeletal muscle. This is most likely the result of

   a. too small a clearance angle
   b. too cold a cryostat temperature
   c. mounting the sections on warm slides
   d. freezing the specimen too slowly

6. The angle formed between the block face and the cutting facet of a knife is known as the:

   a. rake angle
   b. clearance angle
   c. bevel angle
   d. wedge angle

7. Which of the following will most likely be corrected by soaking a faced block in ice water?

   a. lengthwise splits in the sections
   b. compressed and jammed sections
   c. microscopic chatter
   d. mushy sections

8. Which of the following artifacts may be introduced during the flotation process?

   a. holes in the tissue
   b. the "venetian blind" effect
   c. lengthwise splits in the ribbon
   d. separation of tissue elements

9. Which of the following embedding procedures involves first infiltrating the tissue with one medium and then embedding it in another?

   a. double
   b. resin
   c. routine
   d. vacuum

10. A section of liver is cut in the cryostat and the sections obtained are alternately thick and thin, with a distinct "venetian blind" effect. The most probable cause of this artifact is that the:

    a. anti-roll plate is adjusted incorrectly
    b. block is too cold
    c. knife is dull
    d. liver is fatty

11. The type of microtome used for routine paraffin sectioning is a(n):

   a. rotary
   b. sliding
   c. ultramicrotome
   d. retracting

12. When frozen sections stick to a cryostat anti-roll plate, the plate is:

   a. below the knife edge
   b. too warm
   c. not parallel to the knife edge
   d. above the knife edge

13. Knives used for sectioning paraffin blocks should be cleaned with:

   a. alcohol and water
   b. ether and acetone
   c. water and toluene
   d. xylene and alcohol

14. To remove grit and dirt before embedding, paraffin may have to be:

   a. filtered
   b. heated
   c. solidified
   d. washed

15. Microorganism contaminants on slides are usually picked up:

   a. during sectioning
   b. from the staining solution
   c. from the flotation bath
   d. during slide drying

16. When a frozen tissue block rubs the anti-roll plate, the plate is:

   a. too far below the knife edge
   b. defective on the edge
   c. not parallel to the knife edge
   d. too far above the knife edge

17. Microscopic examination of an H&E-stained section reveals the presence of irregular holes scattered throughout the section. This is most likely caused by:

   a. albumin spread on the slide by a finger
   b. excess section adhesive on the slide
   c. sections being taken immediately after "rough facing" of the block
   d. the flotation bath not being cleaned between blocks

18. It is important that the facet of a cryostat knife be small to prevent:

    a. loose metal shavings from attaching to the sections
    b. problems with the anti-roll plate
    c. the section from curling as it is cut
    d. the "venetian blind" effect

19. Multiple skin sections should be embedded with the epithelial surfaces facing in:

    a. one direction
    b. opposite directions
    c. perpendicular directions
    d. random directions

20. Microscopic examination of an H&E-stained section reveals marked background staining. This is most likely caused by:

    a. albumin spread on the slide by a finger
    b. excess section adhesive on the slide
    c. sections being taken immediately after "rough facing" of the block
    d. the flotation bath not being cleaned between blocks

21. Sections of paraffin-embedded tissue show straight lines that appear to be fissures or cuts running at many different angles. This artifact is most likely due to:

    a. improper fixation of the tissue
    b. introduction of water to the block surface
    c. poor gross dissection technique
    d. use of quick-freeze spray to chill the block

22. Hard or bony tissue should be embedded:

    a. parallel to the block edge
    b. on its edge
    c. on its end
    d. at an angle

23. Tubular tissue structures should be embedded:

    a. flat
    b. on edge
    c. on end
    d. parallel to the block edge

24. To protect the exposed tissue during storage, paraffin blocks may need to be:

    a. dipped
    b. filed
    c. stacked
    d. trimmed

25. The edge of a newly-sharpened microtome knife should be checked with a:

    a. dissecting microscope
    b. finger
    c. hair
    d. paper

26. A microtome is the most likely cause of poor sections when the microtome is:

    a. new
    b. placed on an incline
    c. old or has worn surfaces
    d. used by several technicians

27. When frozen sections appear above the anti-roll plate of a cryostat, the plate is:

    a. too warm
    b. too far below the knife edge
    c. defective on the edge
    d. not parallel to the knife edge

28. Biopsies of which of the following tissue should be sectioned at 2 micrometers?

    a. bladder
    b. heart
    c. kidney
    d. liver

29. Which of the following will cause a split or lengthwise scratch in a paraffin ribbon?

    a. debris on the knife edge
    b. inadequate processing
    c. a knife edge that is too sharp
    d. using embedding paraffin with the wrong melting point

30. The purpose of embedding tissue in paraffin is to:

    a. preserve its antigenicity
    b. stabilize proteins
    c. provide support
    d. remove water from the cells

31. Which of the following groups of special stains requires sections cut at 8 to 10 μm?

    a. Congo red, Lieb crystal violet, Bielchowsky
    b. Kinyoun, Snook, Oil red O
    c. von Kossa, Fontana-Masson, Sudan black B
    d. Verhoeff-van Gieson, aldehyde fuchsin, Masson trichrome

32. During sectioning of a block of uterine tissue, alternate thick and thin zones are observed. This is most likely caused by:

   a. improper embedding
   b. inadequate processing
   c. vibration of the knife
   d. non-parallel block edges

33. Microscopic examination of an H&E-stained section reveals the presence of extraneous epithelial cells. This is most likely caused by:

   a. albumin spread on the slide by a finger
   b. excess section adhesive on the slide
   c. sections being taken immediately after "rough facing" of the block
   d. the flotation bath not being cleaned between blocks

34. Disposable knife blades should be discarded:

   a. by incineration
   b. by wrapping with tape and placing in wastepaper basket
   c. in a separate "sharps" box
   d. via the garbage disposal

35. When tissue varies in hardness within a sample, such as skin or bone, the block should be positioned in the microtome so that the:

   a. knife passes through the hardest portion first
   b. knife passes through the hardest portion last
   c. hardest portion is sectioned vertically on the right side
   d. hardest portion has been removed before embedding

36. Of the following tissues, which is should be sectioned at 3 micrometers?

   a. brain
   b. breast
   c. liver
   d. lymph node

37. When frozen sections split vertically as they are cut, the anti-roll plate is:

   a. too warm
   b. too far below the knife edge
   c. defective on the edge
   d. not parallel to the knife edge

38. Which of the following knife profiles is recommended for the majority of paraffin microtomy?

   a. biconcave
   b. planoconcave
   c. tool edge
   d. wedge

39. Lubricants used during knife sharpening are usually composed of:

    a. acid
    b. agar
    c. gelatin
    d. oil

40. The orientation of a specimen for embedding should be decided during:

    a. fixation
    b. grossing
    c. processing
    d. surgical removal

41. When cutting 30 μm sections of fixed brain tissue in a -15°C cryostat, the sections fragment at the knife edge. This problem could most likely be prevented by:

    a. lowering the cryostat temperature to -30°C
    b. raising the cryostat temperature to -5°C
    c. freezing the tissue in liquid nitrogen
    d. using the anti-roll plate

42. Unfixed cryostat sections are most commonly attached to slides by:

    a. placing them in water and then floating onto clean slides
    b. brushing them onto a clean, very cold slide
    c. picking them up from the knife onto an albuminized slide
    d. picking them up from the knife onto a clean, warm slide

43. When paraffin with a 54° to 56°C melting point is used for embedding, the temperature of the flotation bath should fall within which of the following temperature (°C) ranges?

    a. 41 to 45
    b. 46 to 50
    c. 51 to 55
    d. 56 to 60

44. Routine cryostat sections are usually cut at:

    a. -10°C
    b. -20°C
    c. -30°C
    d. -40°C

45. Sections are being lifted from the knife on the upstroke. This is probably because the:

    a. knife is too sharp
    b. knife tilt is incorrect
    c. paraffin is too cold
    d. specimen is too hard

46. Which of the following groups of abrasive compounds is used for microtome knife sharpening?

    a. carborundum, diamond, zinc oxide
    b. diamond, zinc oxide, jeweler's rouge
    c. lead acetate, zinc oxide, jeweler's rouge
    d. carborundum, diamond, jeweler's rouge

47. Cryostat sections of fixed tissue are tending to float off the slides during staining. This problem can be prevented by:

    a. coating the slides with an adhesive mixture
    b. heating the slides over a Bunsen burner
    c. picking up the sections on a room temperature slide
    d. sectioning at a warmer temperature

48. The proper speed for cutting frozen sections:

    a. is fast and even
    b. is slow and even
    c. is similar to that used for paraffin sections
    d. varies with the tissue and temperature

49. The block is faced and sections are cut and mounted on a slide. More of the block is trimmed away and more sections are cut and mounted on a slide. The sections produced by this technique are known as:

    a. consecutives
    b. levels
    c. ribbons
    d. serials

50. To prevent the formation of a thick layer of paraffin on the bottom of the mold during embedding, the tissue must be:

    a. embedded quickly and neatly
    b. handled carefully and slowly
    c. heated directly on a hot plate
    d. reoriented several times

51. The tissue surface to be cut should be placed against which aspect of the embedding mold?

    a. bottom
    b. edge
    c. side
    d. top

52. Paraffin is converted from the fluid state to the solid state by:

    a. crystallization
    b. evaporation
    c. polymerization
    d. sublimation

53. Routine paraffin sections are cut at what micrometer (micron, μm) setting?

    a. 1 to 2
    b. 4 to 5
    c. 7 to 8
    d. 10 to 12

54. As the block face is trimmed, the knife digs into the tissue and gouges out a chunk. The most probable cause of this problem is that the:

    a. block is too cool
    b. knife is dull
    c. block is loose in the chuck
    d. cutting stroke is too rapid

55. Nuclear bubbling is seen on an H&E section. This most likely was caused by:

    a. overfixing the tissue
    b. drying undrained slides at too high a temperature
    c. cutting sections at the wrong micrometer setting
    d. adding adhesive to the flotation bath

56. The clearance angle used with most microtome knives is:

    a. 3 to 8 degrees
    b. 15 to 23 degrees
    c. 27 to 32 degrees
    d. 42 to 45 degrees

57. Microscopic examination of an H&E-stained section reveals the presence of extraneous tumor cells. This is most likely caused by:

    a. albumin spread on the slide by a finger
    b. excess section adhesive on the slide
    c. sections being taken immediately after "rough facing" of the block
    d. the flotation bath not being cleaned between blocks

58. Layered structures such as cyst wall and gallbladder should be embedded:

    a. lengthwise
    b. on edge
    c. on end
    d. parallel to block side

59. During paraffin embedding, it is noted that several sections appear soft and mushy. This is most likely due to:

    a. inadequate processing
    b. prolonged fixation
    c. paraffin that is too warm
    d. the type of tissue processed

60. Which of the following is necessary to ensure a straight ribbon?

    a. horizontal sides of the block must be parallel.
    b. vertical sides of the block must be parallel.
    c. horizontal and vertical sides of the block must be parallel.
    d. the microtome wheel must be rotated rapidly.

61. Microscopic examination of stained slides shows bacilli on, but not in, the tissue sections. The most probable cause of this contaminant is that:

    a. excess albumin on the slides attracted microorganisms
    b. excess gelatin was added to the water bath
    c. the water bath was not cleaned after previous use
    d. there is excess poly-L-lysine on the slides

62. Paraffin used for embedding should be how many degrees centigrade above the melting point of the medium?

    a. 0 to 1
    b. 2 to 4
    c. 5 to 7
    d. 8 to 10

63. Sections of brain that tend to wash off slides during staining can be adhered to slides by coating the section/slide with:

    a. Carbowax™
    b. polyethylene glycol
    c. paraffin
    d. poly-L-lysine

64. Frozen sections are required when:

    a. excellent morphological detail is required
    b. immediate microscopic evaluation is required
    c. demonstration of cytoplasmic IgG is to be done
    d. retinal pathology is suspected

65. When frozen sections partially jam and partially slide under the anti-roll plate, the plate is:

    a. too warm
    b. too far below the knife edge
    c. not parallel to the knife edge
    d. too far above the knife edge

66. One cause of sections sticking to each other or to parts of the microtome is:

    a. air currents
    b. a radio operating in the room
    c. static electricity
    d. the wrong air temperature

67. Microtome knives used for paraffin sectioning are usually made of:

   a. carbon steel
   b. diamond
   c. glass
   d. iron

68. Which of the following groups of plates may be used to support abrasive powders and lubricants for sharpening knives?

   a. copper, glass, and iron
   b. aluminum, copper, and glass
   c. copper, iron, and aluminum
   d. glass, aluminum, and iron

69. Which of the following problems will be seen in paraffin sections that are floated out on a flotation bath that is too cold?

   a. cracks
   b. folds
   c. separations
   d. stretching

70. During microtomy, several successive paraffin sections are compressed and wrinkled. The most appropriate action is to:

   a. change to a new blade
   b. increase the rapidity of cutting
   c. check the paraffin melting point
   d. increase the flotation bath temperature

71. Refer to the following data:

   Cryostat Temperature Chart

Day	Temperature (°C)
Monday	-20
Tuesday	-15
Wednesday	-18
Thursday	-23
Friday	-26

   On which day would sectioning of breast tissue be most difficult?

   a. Monday
   b. Tuesday
   c. Thursday
   d. Friday

72. Which of the following could be substituted for gelatin as an additive to the flotation bath?

   a. aminoalkylsilane
   b. chromium potassium sulfate
   c. poly-L-lysine
   d. agar

73. During microtomy, it is noted that a faced block that has been soaking in ice water contains a bulging white area. This is most likely the result of:

   a. the presence of suture material
   b. incomplete decalcification
   c. prolonged fixation
   d. inadequate dehydration

74. Lymph node tissue shatters when sectioned in a cryostat maintained at -20°C. The most appropriate action is to:

   a. switch to an unused part of the knife
   b. increase the knife tilt
   c. chill the block with a spray coolant
   d. warm the block slightly

75. For good demonstration of myelin sheaths, paraffin sections should be:

   a. floated on a cool water bath
   b. cut 10 to 15 μm thick
   c. coated with celloidin
   d. dried at room temperature

76. In paraffin microtomy, knowledge of the possible disease process present in the tissue may be important because it may change the requirements in:

   a. clearance angle
   b. section thickness
   c. flotation medium
   d. knife temperature

77. Prominent peripheral chatter is obtained on sections of a paraffin block that has been routinely fixed and processed. This can probably be corrected by recutting the block:

   a. after soaking it in ice water
   b. using a faster cutting speed
   c. after re-embedding in a different paraffin
   d. using a greater clearance angle

78. Slides used for mounting open-top cryostat frozen sections should be kept at the same temperature as the:

a. tissue
b. knife
c. operator
d. room

79. Paraffin sections should be cut at 2 micrometers when studying:

a. basement membranes
b. myelin
c. amyloid
d. nerve fibers

80. The tissue block fails to advance during the preparation of frozen sections. This probably could be corrected by:

a. changing the knife angle
b. replacing the knife
c. decreasing the chamber temperature
d. cleaning and oiling the microtome

81. An H&E-stained lymph node section reveals overlapping nuclei. This indicates that the section is most likely:

a. overstained with hematoxylin
b. too thick
c. of an abnormal node
d. appropriately sectioned

82. The material of choice for immunofluorescence microscopy and enzyme histochemical studies is:

a. paraffin sections
b. cryostat sections
c. air-dried imprints
d. alcohol-fixed imprints

83. When a femoral head is sectioned, the marrow portion sections satisfactorily but the cortex fragments. The most probable cause of this problem is that the:

a. decalcifying agent was too strong
b. embedding medium is too hard
c. decalcifying agent was not washed out
d. compact bone is underdecalcified

84. A fingernail has been fixed in formalin, routinely processed, and embedded in paraffin. The tissue is very hard and sections are difficult to obtain. Sectioning quality will be improved and tissue components will be best preserved and demonstrated by gently facing the block and:

   a. soaking in water
   b. warming the block slightly
   c. soaking in a solution that softens keratin
   d. treating with a decalcifying fluid

The following items (*) have been identified as more appropriate for entry-level histotechnologists.

* 85 The solution used in the knife trough when sectioning epoxy resins is usually:

   a. dioxane
   b. EDTA
   c. water
   d. xylene

* 86. The shape of the face of a trimmed resin block should be a:

   a. parallelogram
   b. rectangle
   c. square
   d. trapezoid

* 87. A section of skeletal muscle has been frozen in isopentane and liquid nitrogen, but numerous holes are seen in the H&E-stained sections. This problem is most commonly caused by:

   a. non-isometrically fixed muscle tissue
   b. sectioning too soon after freezing
   c. leaving in the isopentane too long
   d. isopentane that is not cold enough

* 88. "Thick" sections for electron microscopy, or sections to be viewed with the light microscope, are cut at:

   a. 4 to 6 nanometers
   b. 60 to 70 nanometers
   c. 0.5 to 1.0 micrometers
   d. 4 to 6 micrometers

* 89. A diamond knife should NOT be used to cut tissue containing:

   a. amyloid
   b. calcium
   c. lipid
   d. erythrocytes

* 90. The ultrathin resin sections best suited for electron microscopy appear as what color when viewed with fluorescent light through the binocular microscope?

   a. blue
   b. purple
   c. silver
   d. yellow

* 91. Tissues to be sectioned with a cryostat may be somewhat protected from ice crystal artifacts by:

   a. chilling in the refrigerator before freezing
   b. freezing the tissue very slowly
   c. using gum tragacanth to mount the tissue on the object disc
   d. infiltrating with 30% sucrose before freezing

* 92. The surface of the liquid in the trough of a glass knife should be:

   a. concave
   b. convex
   c. horizontal
   d. vertical

* 93. A section of skeletal muscle has been frozen in isopentane and liquid nitrogen, but numerous holes are seen in the H&E-stained sections. This problem might be prevented in the future by:

   a. freezing in liquid nitrogen alone
   b. sectioning immediately after freezing
   c. making sure that the isopentane is at -150°C
   d. isometrically fixing the section of muscle

* 94. During the sectioning of plastic blocks with an ultramicrotome, no sections are visible in the trough. The problem is most likely caused by:

   a. dirt
   b. a dull knife
   c. a loose knife
   d. an incorrect water level

* 95. Glass knives suitable for cutting plastic blocks of medium hardness will have a cutting edge angle of:

   a. 25°
   b. 35°
   c. 45°
   d. 55°

* 96. During the sectioning of plastic blocks with an ultramicrotome, no sections are being cut. The problem is most likely caused by:

   a. dirt
   b. a dull knife
   c. a loose knife
   d. an incorrect water level

* 97. During the sectioning of plastic blocks with an ultramicrotome, scratches are seen in the sections. The problem is most likely caused by:

   a. dirt
   b. a dull knife
   c. a loose knife
   d. an incorrect water level

* 98. The microtome used for electron microscopy is called a(n):

   a. rotary microtome
   b. sliding microtome
   c. freezing microtome
   d. ultramicrotome

* 99. During the sectioning of plastic blocks with an ultramicrotome, the sections are sticking to the block. The problem is most likely caused by:

   a. dirt
   b. a dull knife
   c. a loose knife
   d. an incorrect water level

* 100. Sections MUST be mounted onto coated grids for viewing with an electron microscope if they have been embedded in:

   a. Araldite™
   b. celloidin
   c. Epon™
   d. methacrylate

* 101. Resin sections are remaining compressed when floated on the water in the trough of the diamond knife. To aid in expanding the sections, a strip of paper dipped in which of the following may be waved over the section?

   a. acetic acid
   b. formalin
   c. dioxane
   d. chloroform

* 102. Glass knives are being made for cutting ultrathin sections. The time limit for obtaining good sections requires that these knives should be used within the same ___ as being made:

a. hour
b. day
c. week
d. month

* 103. During the sectioning of plastic blocks with an ultramicrotome, alternating thick and thin sections are obtained. The problem is most likely caused by:

a. dirt
b. a dull knife
c. a loose knife
d. an incorrect water level

* 104. The type of knife most frequently used to cut ultrathin sections for electron microscopy is:

a. aluminum
b. diamond
c. glass
d. stainless steel

* 105. Passing a gloved finger over the surface of frozen tissue to raise its temperature is contraindicated for tissues being sectioned for the demonstration of:

a. carbohydrates
b. enzymes
c. glycogen
d. mucins

* 106. Diamond knives are used in ultramicrotomy because steel knives:

a. cannot withstand the electron beam
b. leave steel shavings in ultra-thin sections
c. react with the chemicals in the resin blocks
d. are quickly dulled

* 107. "Thin" sections for viewing with electron microscopy are cut at:

a. 4 to 6 nanometers
b. 60 to 70 nanometers
c. 0.6 to 0.7 micrometers
d. 6 to 7 micrometers

* 108. Grids used to support epoxy-embedded sections for electron microscopy are usually made from:

    a. copper
    b. iron
    c. lead
    d. zinc

* 109. Undecalcified bone can be sectioned most easily when embedded in:

    a. celloidin
    b. plastic
    c. water soluble wax
    d. paraffin

* 110. Sections of epoxy-embedded kidney contain vertical streaks through the entire section. This most likely was caused by:

    a. the wrong knife angle
    b. poor infiltration
    c. imperfections in the knife edge
    d. unpolymerized resin

* 111. A technician is having trouble getting all paraffin-embedded blocks to ribbon. Examination reveals that the tissues were embedded in 62°C melting-point paraffin and the room temperature is 25°C. Which of the following actions should correct the problem in the future?

    a. immediately ordering some lower melting point paraffin
    b. soaking faced blocks in ice water before ribboning
    c. warming faced blocks before ribboning
    d. lowering the room temperature

* 112. The instrumentation QC manual states that flotation baths must be emptied and thoroughly cleaned on Fridays. The bath may be refilled and additional adhesive may be added as needed during the week. This procedure:

    a. may be considered as satisfactory
    b. should be changed to read "emptied and cleaned twice a week"
    c. may lead to bacterial contamination of microscopic sections
    d. will probably increase section loss during staining

* 113. Periodic acid methenamine-silver (PAMS)-stained kidney sections reveal well-impregnated basement membranes. However, within the individual glomeruli the membranes overlap and cannot be evaluated as separate structures. This could be corrected by cutting sections at:

    a. 2 to 3 micrometers
    b. 5 to 6 micrometers
    c. 8 to 9 micrometers
    d. 13 to 15 micrometers

* 114. A microscopic section of liver tissue shows numerous irregular holes throughout the tissue. This is most likely because:

    a. the holes are portal triads
    b. liver is difficult to cut
    c. fixation has been prolonged
    d. sectioning technique was poor

* 115. A student is having difficulty cutting Carbowax™-embedded tissue using the following technique:
    - chilling the block with ice
    - sectioning at 5 microns with a slow cutting speed
    - placing the sections directly on the slide
    - drying at 45°C
    - staining with H&E

    The problem would most likely be solved by:

    a. floating sections on a water bath
    b. not chilling the block with ice
    c. cutting thinner sections
    d. sectioning at a faster cutting speed

* 116. Successive cryostat sections catch on one area in the middle of the anti-roll plate. The most likely cause is that the anti-roll plate is:

    a. warmer than the knife
    b. colder than the knife
    c. improperly adjusted
    d. damaged

* 117. Mayer egg albumin is observed to be contaminated with bacterial growth. The most probable explanation is that during preparation:

    a. the reagent was inadequately heated
    b. a non-sterile storage container was used
    c. thymol was omitted
    d. the eggs used in preparation were contaminated

* 118. A ribbon of paraffin-embedded brain tissue is floated on the water bath. Small holes are noted in the first section that decrease in size in subsequent sections. The most appropriate action is to:

    a. melt the block and re-embed the tissue
    b. resharpen the knife
    c. decrease the water bath temperature
    d. cut and discard ribbons until the holes disappear

* 119. Breathing on blocks during sectioning should be kept to a minimum when using:

    a. celloidin
    b. Epon™
    c. paraffin wax
    d. polyester wax

Microtomy Answer Key

The following items have been identified as appropriate for both entry level histologic technicians and histotechnologists.

1. b	22. d	43. b	64. b
2. c	23. c	44. b	65. c
3. a	24. a	45. b	66. c
4. a	25. a	46. d	67. a
5. d	26. c	47. a	68. a
6. b	27. b	48. c	69. b
7. c	28. c	49. b	70. a
8. d	29. a	50. a	71. b
9. a	30. c	51. a	72. d
10. c	31. a	52. a	73. d
11. a	32. c	53. b	74. d
12. b	33. a	54. c	75. b
13. d	34. c	55. b	76. b
14. a	35. b	56. a	77. a
15. c	36. d	57. d	78. d
16. d	37. c	58. b	79. a
17. c	38. d	59. a	80. d
18. b	39. d	60. a	81. b
19. a	40. b	61. c	82. b
20. b	41. b	62. b	83. d
21. d	42. d	63. d	84. c

The following items (*) have been identified as more appropriate for the entry level histotechnologists.

* 85. c	* 94. d	* 103. c	* 112. c
* 86. d	* 95. c	* 104. b	* 113. a
* 87. d	* 96. b	* 105. b	* 114. d
* 88. c	* 97. a	* 106. d	* 115. b
* 89. b	* 98. d	* 107. b	* 116. d
* 90. c	* 99. d	* 108. a	* 117. c
* 91. d	* 100. d	* 109. b	* 118. d
* 92. a	* 101. d	* 110. c	* 119. d
* 93. c	* 102. b	* 111. a	

Chapter 12

Processing

The following items have been identified as appropriate for both entry-level histologic technicians and histotechnologists.

1. During microtomy, it is noted that many of the tissues to be examined seem very hard and shrunken. Of the following, the most likely explanation for this problem is that the:

   a. infiltrating paraffin is too hot
   b. processing reagents need changing
   c. pH of the fixative was incorrect
   d. clearing agent is contaminated with water

2. Decalcification of small specimens can be achieved by fixation in:

   a. neutral buffered formalin
   b. Zenker solution
   c. glutaraldehyde
   d. Zamboni solution

3. A major disadvantage of aliphatic clearing agents is that they:

   a. are incompatible with some mounting media
   b. have a very high penetration rate
   c. harden tissue excessively
   d. are highly toxic

4. Which of the following is MOST likely to cause sensitization with prolonged use?

   a. cedarwood oil
   b. xylene
   c. aliphatic hydrocarbons
   d. limonene

5. To speed up the laboratory's processing of all surgical tissues, the temperature of all fixation, dehydration, and clearing steps has been set at 45°C. This will most likely result in:

    a. excellent sections of all tissue
    b. very soft uterine scrapings
    c. overprocessed biopsy tissue
    d. sections that will not stain with eosin

6. Limonene functions as a(n):

    a. clearing agent only
    b. dehydrating agent only
    c. universal solvent
    d. infiltrating medium

7. One advantage of aliphatic hydrocarbons is that they:

    a. have a high tolerance for water
    b. are miscible with all mounting media
    c. are low in toxicity and sensitization
    d. are adaptable to various processing methods

8. A disadvantage of using heat at all stations of the enclosed tissue processor is that it will:

    a. harden some tissues
    b. lengthen processing time
    c. shorten the processor lifespan
    d. cause too much reagent evaporation

9. Dehydration refers to the removal of:

    a. alcohol
    b. paraffin
    c. water
    d. xylene

10. Which decalcification method may cause burning of the specimen?

    a. acid
    b. chelation
    c. electrolytic
    d. ion-exchange

11. Which of the following clearing agents is NOT flammable?

    a. benzene
    b. chloroform
    c. toluene
    d. xylene

12. Which of the following groups of reagents may be used for dehydration?

    a. ethanol, limonene, and tetrahydrofuran
    b. methanol, ethanol, and limonene
    c. dioxane, methanol, and toluene
    d. dioxane, methanol, and ethanol

13. Which of the following is routinely used in electron microscopy?

    a. agar
    b. celloidin
    c. ester wax
    d. resin

14. A clearing agent must be miscible with:

    a. dehydrants and infiltrating media
    b. fixatives and dehydrants
    c. fixatives and infiltrating media
    d. universal solvents

15. Which of the following is a chelating agent used for decalcification?

    a. ethylenediaminetetraacetic acid
    b. hydrochloric acid
    c. trichloracetic acid
    d. phenol

16. The alcohols on the automated tissue processor should be changed on a regular basis because:

    a. the alcohols become saturated with bile from gall bladder specimens, which can be absorbed by other tissues
    b. too great a concentration of formalin in the alcohols can create a potentially explosive situation
    c. gram-negative organisms can start growing in alcohol left too long on the tissue processor
    d. the alcohols can absorb moisture and become dilute

17. After completion of decalcification, the specimen should be:

    a. placed in acetone
    b. rinsed with 70% alcohol
    c. transferred to fixative
    d. washed in water

18. Which of the processing schedules shown below should be used to process fixed routine surgical tissue in a closed processor?

Schedule A		Schedule B		Schedule C	
Formol-alcohol	2 hrs	80% alcohol	20 min	80% alcohol	8 hrs
95% alcohol	1 hr	80% alcohol	20 min	95% alcohol	4 hrs
95% alcohol	1 hr	95% alcohol	20 min	95% alcohol	4 hrs
Abs. alcohol	1 hr	95% alcohol	20 min	Abs. alcohol	4 hrs
Abs. alcohol	1 hr	Abs. alcohol	20 min	Abs. alcohol	4 hrs
Xylene	1 hr	Abs. alcohol	20 min	Chloroform	1 hr
Xylene	1 hr	Abs. alcohol	20 min	Chloroform	1 hr
Paraffin	1 hr	Xylene	20 min	Chloroform	1 hr
Paraffin	1 hr	Xylene	20 min	Paraffin	2 hrs
Paraffin	1 hr	Paraffin	20 min	Paraffin	2 hrs
Paraffin	20 min	Paraffin	20 min	Paraffin	2 hrs

a. Schedule A
b. Schedule B
c. Schedule C
d. none of the above is adequate

19. Ethanol functions as a(n):

a. dehydrating agent
b. clearing agent
c. universal solvent
d. infiltrating medium

20. Which of the processing schedules shown below should be used to process a fixed-needle biopsy of the liver using a closed tissue processor?

Schedule A		Schedule B		Schedule C	
Formol-alcohol	2 hrs	80% alcohol	20 min	80% alcohol	8 hrs
95% alcohol	1 hr	80% alcohol	20 min	95% alcohol	4 hrs
95% alcohol	1 hr	95% alcohol	20 min	95% alcohol	4 hrs
Abs. alcohol	1 hr	95% alcohol	20 min	Abs. alcohol	4 hrs
Abs. alcohol	1 hr	Abs. alcohol	20 min	Abs. alcohol	4 hrs
Xylene	1 hr	Abs. alcohol	20 min	Chloroform	1 hr
Xylene	1 hr	Abs. alcohol	20 min	Chloroform	1 hr
Paraffin	1 hr	Xylene	20 min	Chloroform	1 hr
Paraffin	1 hr	Xylene	20 min	Paraffin	2 hrs
Paraffin	1 hr	Paraffin	20 min	Paraffin	2 hrs
Paraffin	20 min	Paraffin	20 min	Paraffin	2 hrs

a. Schedule A
b. Schedule B
c. Schedule C
d. none of the above is adequate

21. Butyl alcohol is recommended as a dehydrant for:

a. blood smears
b. brain tissue
c. plant tissue
d. spleen

22. Isopropanol functions as a(n):

a. dehydrating agent only
b. clearing agent only
c. universal solvent
d. infiltrating medium

23. Dehydrating tissues in graded alcohols of increasing concentrations is superior to using absolute alcohol only because it will:

a. cause less distortion of the tissue
b. be less harmful to the tissue processor
c. not harden tissue over a long period
d. remove the fixative faster

24. When preparing tissues for electron microscopy, the degree of dehydration should be:

   a. partial
   b. complete
   c. unrelated to subsequent steps
   d. different for each embedding medium

25. The best method of preparing tissue for enzyme demonstration is:

   a. agar embedding
   b. celloidin embedding
   c. paraffin embedding
   d. unfixed frozen sections

26. Glycol methacrylate functions as a(n):

   a. dehydrating agent only
   b. clearing agent only
   c. universal solvent
   d. infiltrating medium

27. Fat remains in the tissue following infiltration with:

   a. Carbowax™
   b. celloidin
   c. paraffin
   d. glycol methacrylate

28. Methanol functions as a(n):

   a. dehydrating agent only
   b. clearing agent only
   c. universal solvent
   d. infiltrating medium

29. The most rapid-freezing tissue is the result of using:

   a. aerosol sprays
   b. dry ice
   c. gaseous carbon dioxide
   d. liquid nitrogen/isopentane

30. The amount of time a specimen needs to remain in decalcifying solution is NOT influenced by the:

   a. bone density
   b. processing schedule
   c. solution strength
   d. solution temperature

31. Tissue will NOT be damaged by extended periods of time in:

   a. acetone
   b. benzene
   c. cedarwood oil
   d. absolute ethanol

32. Tissue must be dehydrated before placing it in:

   a. agar
   b. Carbowax™
   c. Epon™
   d. gelatin

33. Which of the following chemicals can be used to indicate the presence of water in alcohol?

   a. copper sulfite
   b. copper sulfate
   c. sodium sulfite
   d. sodium sulfate

34. The ideal thickness of specimens to be decalcified is:

   a. 1 to 2 mm
   b. 3 to 4 mm
   c. 6 to 7 mm
   d. 9 to 10 mm

35. Paraffin processing is contraindicated for the subsequent demonstration of:

   a. enzymes
   b. mucins
   c. nuclei
   d. proteins

36. Which of the following reagents is miscible with water, alcohol, hydrocarbons, and paraffin?

   a. acetone
   b. cedarwood oil
   c. dioxane
   d. xylene

37. When using epoxy resins during processing, which of the following is typically used as the transitional fluid between alcohol and the epoxy resin?

   a. acetone
   b. chloroform
   c. dioxane
   d. propylene oxide

38. Refer to the schedule shown below. If processing starts at 12 noon, in which solution will the tissue be at 1:45 pm?

Schedule

80% alcohol	20 min
80% alcohol	20 min
95% alcohol	20 min
95% alcohol	20 min
Abs. alcohol	20 min
Abs. alcohol	20 min ✓
Abs. alcohol	20 min
Xylene	20 min
Xylene	20 min
Paraffin	20 min
Paraffin	20 min
Paraffin	2 hrs

a. first absolute alcohol
b. second absolute alcohol
c. third absolute alcohol
d. first xylene

39. Prolonged dehydration in higher grades of alcohol will render a specimen:

a. hard
b. macerated
c. porous
d. toxic

40. For adequate clearing in xylene during routine processing, tissue should have a maximum thickness of:

a. 1 to 2 mm
b. 3 to 4 mm
c. 5 to 6 mm
d. 7 to 8 mm

41. Cedarwood oil functions as a(n):

a. dehydrating agent only
b. clearing agent only
c. universal solvent
d. infiltrating medium

42. Processing of delicate tissues (eg, embryonic tissues) should be started in what concentration of alcohol?

a. 30%
b. 50%
c. 70%
d. 90%

43. Chloroform functions as a(n):

a. dehydrating agent only
b. clearing agent only
c. universal solvent
d. infiltrating medium

44. The effect of overdecalcification is most noticeable in the staining of:

a. nuclei
b. cytoplasm
c. erythrocytes
d. bone spicules

45. Which of the following is considered to always be the best dehydrant?

a. acetone
b. ethanol
c. isopropanol
d. methanol

46. All of the following are methods for checking the completeness of decalcification EXCEPT:

a. chemical
b. electrolytic
c. mechanical
d. radiographic

47. Acid solutions soften bone tissue by removing which of the following salts?

a. calcium
b. lithium
c. potassium
d. sodium

48. A process that can preserve enzymes and prevent the loss of some cellular constituents is:

a. autoradiography
b. freeze-drying
c. infiltration
d. vaporization

49. If the clearing agent is cloudy, it may be contaminated with:

    a. absolute alcohol
    b. bacteria
    c. water
    d. yeast

50. Dioxane functions as a(n):

    a. dehydrating agent only
    b. clearing agent only
    c. universal solvent
    d. infiltrating medium

51. Which of the following gases is released during decalcification?

    a. ammonia
    b. carbon dioxide
    c. nitrous oxide
    d. oxygen

52. Epon™ functions as a(n):

    a. dehydrating agent only
    b. clearing agent only
    c. universal solvent
    d. infiltrating medium

53. Tetrahydrofuran functions as a(n):

    a. dehydrating agent only
    b. clearing agent only
    c. universal solvent
    d. infiltrating medium

54. During processing for electron microscopy, specimen dehydration using absolute ethanol should be carried out in capped vials because when specimens are left open there is a tendency for:

    a. air bubbles to form
    b. oxidation artifacts to form
    c. solution precipitation to occur
    d. absorption of atmospheric moisture

55. The time needed for infiltration of paraffin into a tissue specimen is dependent upon all of the following EXCEPT the:

    a. fixative used
    b. thickness of the specimen
    c. tissue type
    d. use of vacuum

56. Xylene functions as a(n):

    a. dehydrating agent
    b. clearing agent
    c. universal solvent
    d. infiltrating medium

57. To offset the hydrolysis of nucleic acids caused by decalcifying agents, bone marrow biopsy specimens are sometimes fixed in:

    a. buffered formalin
    b. glutaraldehyde
    c. osmium tetroxide
    d. Zenker solution

58. Which of the following can be used to hold exudate or friable tissues in place for processing?

    a. agar
    b. celloidin
    c. paraffin
    d. resin

59. The longest time that tissues can remain in cedarwood oil without any apparent harm is:

    a. minutes
    b. hours
    c. days
    d. months

60. Decalcification occurs with all of the following methods EXCEPT:

    a. simple acid
    b. radiographic
    c. chelation
    d. ion-exchange

61. Which of the following is soluble in various fat solvents?

    a. agar
    b. Carbowax™
    c. gelatin
    d. paraffin

62. The process of saturating tissue with the medium that will be used for embedding is called:

    a. clearing
    b. dehydration
    c. fixation
    d. infiltration

63. Toluene functions as a(n):

   a. dehydrating agent only
   b. clearing agent only
   c. universal solvent
   d. infiltrating medium

64. Of the reagents listed below, the best substitute for ethanol for processing tissues is:

   a. dioxane
   b. butanol
   c. isopropanol
   d. methanol

65. Refer to the schedule shown below. If processing is started at 8:00 am Monday, at what time on Tuesday will the tissue be ready to embed?

   Schedule

80% alcohol	8 hrs
95% alcohol	4 hrs
95% alcohol	4 hrs
Abs. alcohol	4 hrs
Abs. alcohol	4 hrs
Chloroform	1 hr
Chloroform	1 hr
Chloroform	1 hr
Paraffin	2 hrs
Paraffin	2 hrs
Paraffin	2 hrs (in vacuum)

   a. 4:00 p.m.
   b. 5:00 p.m.
   c. 6:00 p.m.
   d. 7:00 p.m.

66. Which clearing agent must be removed with a volatile hydrocarbon prior to impregnation?

   a. cedarwood oil
   b. carbon bisulfide
   c. carbon tetrachloride
   d. chloroform

67. Which of the following must one do when using an essential oil as a clearing agent?

    a. avoid the use of ethyl alcohol
    b. remove the oil with xylene
    c. avoid exposure to heat
    d. avoid lengthy exposure

68. Slow freezing of tissues prior to sectioning will most likely:

    a. make sectioning difficult
    b. yield sections showing tissue disruption
    c. require a change in the knife clearance angle
    d. preserve antigenic sites

69. An open tissue processor malfunctions, advancing tissue one step further than normal at the end of processing and placing the tissue in fixative. The best course of action is to:

    a. treat the tissue with absolute ethanol, xylene, and then paraffin
    b. embed the tissue without further processing
    c. place the tissue in paraffin for 2 hours, then embed
    d. rehydrate the tissue in saline

70. Determining the end-point of decalcification is very important because:

    a. calcium remaining in the tissue interferes with staining
    b. underdecalcification causes processing problems
    c. overdecalcification results in destruction of cell structure
    d. prolonged acid treatment inhibits good fixation

71. Paraffin with a melting point of 55°C is used for impregnation and embedding. The temperature of the paraffin containers should be regulated at approximately:

    a. 50°C
    b. 55°C
    c. 58°C
    d. 62°C

72. For successful impregnation of tissue, the time needed for infiltration with paraffin depends on the:

    a. melting point of the paraffin
    b. thickness and texture of the tissue
    c. choice of dehydrating agent
    d. the fixative used

* 73. A technologist in the electron microscopy laboratory has developed dermatitis. This problem can most likely be prevented in the future by ensuring that:

    a. a chemical hood is used for processing
    b. the secondary fixation step is eliminated
    c. another resin is selected for embedding
    d. protective gear is worn during processing

* 74. Smudgy nuclei and variations in staining are noted on routinely processed, formalin-fixed colon biopsy specimens. One cause of these problems could be:

    a. overfixation
    b. incomplete dehydration
    c. poor choice of fixative
    d. prolonged clearing

* 75. Processed tissue that was fixed in zinc-formalin is very hard and brittle. The stained sections show microscopic chatter. This problem might be corrected in the future by:

    a. leaving the tissue in the fixative for less than 4 hours
    b. treating the tissue for removal of pigment
    c. placing the tissue in a buffer solution after fixation
    d. selecting a better schedule for processing

* 76. A technologist in the electron microscopy laboratory has developed dermatitis. This is probably because of exposure to:

    a. osmium tetroxide
    b. absolute ethanol
    c. epoxy resin
    d. the electron beam

* 77. When placed in a solution whose refractive index is similar to the refractive index of tissue proteins, tissue becomes:

   a. fragile
   b. hard
   c. small
   d. translucent

* 78. Microscopic review of H&E-stained sections of a colon biopsy show very uneven staining of the tissue and poor nuclear detail. Of the following, the most likely cause is that the:

   a. paraffin block was cooled too slowly
   b. tissue remained in alcohol too long
   c. pH of the fixative was incorrect
   d. clearing agent is contaminated with water

* 79. Xylene, toluene, and benzene belong to what chemical class?

   a. hydrocarbon
   b. ketone
   c. phenol
   d. sterol

* 80. To help preserve membranes in frozen sections, prior to freezing fixed tissue may be placed in a solution of:

   a. gum mastic
   b. saline
   c. sucrose
   d. talc

* 81. Consider the viscosity (in centipoises) at 20°C of the various solutions given below. Which of the solutions would clear most quickly?

   a. benzene (.65)
   b. butanol (2.95)
   c. toluene (.59)
   d. xylene (.7)

* 82. The penetration of any solution into tissue is increased as which of the following is increased?

   a. molecular size of the solution
   b. temperature of the solution
   c. viscosity of the solution
   d. specific gravity of the solution

* 83. To best demonstrate muscle enzymes, which freezing method should be used?

   a. cryostat freezer plate
   b. dry ice
   c. liquid nitrogen
   d. isopentane, pre-chilled to -160°C

* 84. Which of the following groups of chemical families are commonly used as clearing agents?

    a. acetates, aldehydes, chlorinated hydrocarbons, terpenes
    b. alcohols, aromatic hydrocarbons, glycol ethers, methacrylates
    c. aliphatic hydrocarbons, aromatic hydrocarbons, chlorinated hydrocarbons, terpenes
    d. aldehydes, aliphatic hydrocarbons, aromatic hydrocarbons, methacrylates

* 85. Polyethylene glycol is employed as the embedding medium for the preservation of:

    a. enzymes
    b. urate crystals
    c. lipids
    d. keratin

* 86. Araldite™ functions as a(n):

    a. dehydrating agent only
    b. clearing agent only
    c. universal solvent
    d. infiltrating medium

* 87. Consider the viscosity (in centipoises) at 20°C of various solutions given below. Which of the solutions would dehydrate most quickly?

    a. acetone (.3)
    b. ethanol (1.2)
    c. isopropanol (2.5)
    d. methanol (.6)

* 88. Consider the viscosity (in centipoises) at 20°C of the various solutions given below. Which would dehydrate most slowly?

    a. acetone (.3)
    b. ethanol (1.2)
    c. isopropanol (2.5)
    d. methanol (.6)

*89. Consider the viscosity (in centipoises) at 20°C of various solutions given below. Which of the following solutions would clear most slowly?

    a. acetone (.3)
    b. benzene (.65)
    c. toluene (.59)
    d. xylene (.7)

* 90. An alcohol is a compound in which one or more of the hydrogen atoms of a hydrocarbon has been replaced by which of the following groups?

    a. hydroxyl
    b. ketone
    c. methyl
    d. carboxyl

* 91. When processing with water-soluble wax, tissue is fixed, washed with water, and:

a. dehydrated with 95% and absolute alcohols, cleared with xylene, and then infiltrated
b. dehydrated with 95% alcohol and then infiltrated
c. dehydrated and cleared with a universal solvent and then infiltrated
d. infiltrated only

* 92. Which of the following should be selected when tissue must be embedded in a medium that will tolerate a small amount of water?

a. glycol methacrylate
b. celloidin
c. Epon™
d. paraffin

* 93. If a laboratory ran out of ethanol, which of the following dehydrants might be available and suitable for emergency use?

a. dioxane
b. tetrahydrofuran
c. isopropanol
d. butanol

* 94. A lecture includes a discussion of glass knives, epoxy resins, and lead citrate staining. The subject would most likely be:

a. electron microscopy
b. undecalcified bone
c. 1 micron resin sections
d. immunohistochemistry

* 95. High-resolution light microscopy is needed on a lymph node biopsy. To achieve the best results, the specimen should be processed for embedding in:

a. water-soluble wax
b. celloidin
c. glycol methacrylate
d. microcrystalline wax

* 96. A section of kidney is fixed in phosphate-buffered formalin and then routinely processed with 95% alcohol, absolute alcohol, xylene, and paraffin. When sectioned, many vertical knife lines are noted in the sections, and these lines remain in the same area of the tissue even when the knife is moved. This is most likely due to:

a. precipitated phosphates in the tissue
b. defects in the knife edge
c. excessive dehydration of the tissue
d. poor fixation

* 97. Carbowax™ has a major disadvantage of:

a. dissolving during flotation
b. being a lengthy processing method
c. making tissues brittle for sectioning
d. causing cell shrinkage

* 98. Paraffin infiltration at 70°C would:

a. make tissue easier to section
b. preserve lipids better
c. shorten infiltration time by 50%
d. denature tissue antigens

* 99. An oil red O stain has been requested on a friable specimen that must be embedded for sectioning. The embedding medium that should be used is:

a. plastic
b. paraffin
c. water-soluble wax
d. celloidin

* 100. Carbowax™ is soluble in:

a. water
b. benzene
c. xylene
d. ether

* 101. While performing the daily temperature check of the embedding center paraffin reservoir, it is noted that the temperature is 12° above the melting point of paraffin. The most appropriate action is to:

a. drain and replace the paraffin
b. check the thermostat setting
c. recheck the temperature in 24 hours
d. do nothing; the temperature is acceptable

* 102. A method of decalcification is needed for research bone specimens on which subsequent oxidative enzyme stains are essential. Which of the following decalcifying methods should be selected?

a. electrolytic
b. ion-exchange
c. chelating agents
d. simple acid

* 103. Consider a tissue sectioning procedure that must be done with the following specifications:

- contact with water must be avoided in sectioning
- there must be minimum distortion of tissue
- fat stains can be done on the sections
- procedure may require several hours

To which of the following processing techniques do these specifications refer?
a. resin
b. celloidin
c. paraffin
d. water-soluble wax

* 104. In the electrolytic method of decalcification, the specimen to be decalcified is attached to the anode. The reason for this is that:

    a. calcium ions will become neutralized at this site
    b. proteins are more readily neutralized at this site
    c. insoluble calcium salts will form on the anode
    d. calcium ions will migrate to the cathode

* 105. During embedding, tissue is noted to be soft and spongy. The most cost-effective action to prevent this problem from recurring is to:

    a. take hydrometer readings of all alcohols
    b. replace all alcohols and clearing reagents
    c. change the clearing reagent
    d. change all the reagents

* 106. To achieve the best high-resolution light microscopy, specimens should be processed for embedding in:

    a. water-soluble wax
    b. celloidin
    c. glycol methacrylate
    d. paraffin

Processing Answer Key

The following items have been identified as appropriate for both entry level histologic technicians and histotechnologists.

1. a	19. a	37. d	55. a
2. b	20. b	38. b	56. b
3. a	21. c	39. a	57. d
4. d	22. a	40. b	58. a
5. c	23. a	41. b	59. d
6. a	24. b	42. a	60. b
7. c	25. d	43. b	61. d
8. a	26. d	44. a	62. d
9. c	27. a	45. b	63. b
10. c	28. a	46. b	64. c
11. b	29. d	47. a	65. b
12. d	30. b	48. b	66. a
13. d	31. c	49. c	67. b
14. a	32. c	50. c	68. b
15. a	33. b	51. b	69. a
16. d	34. b	52. d	70. c
17. d	35. a	53. c	71. c
18. a	36. c	54. d	72. b

The following items (*) have been identified as more appropriate for the entry level histotechnologists.

* 73. d	* 82. b	* 91. d	* 100. a
* 74. b	* 83. d	* 92. a	* 101. b
* 75. d	* 84. c	* 93. c	* 102. c
* 76. c	* 85. c	* 94. a	* 103. d
* 77. d	* 86. d	* 95. c	* 104. d
* 78. d	* 87. a	* 96. a	* 105. a
* 79. a	* 88. c	* 97. a	* 106. c
* 80. c	* 89. d	* 98. d	
* 81. c	* 90. a	* 99. c	

Chapter 13

Staining

The following items have been identified as appropriate for both entry-level histologic technicians and histotechnologists.

1. When using the Fite procedure, mycobacteria are stained:

   a. blue
   b. orange
   c. red
   d. green

2. Which of the following will bind to acid mucosubstances and may then be demonstrated by the Prussian blue reaction?

   a. diastase
   b. dimedone
   c. colloidal iron
   d. hyaluronidase

3. Parallel sections are stained with PAS, one with and one without diastase digestion. When the staining results are evaluated, the digested section demonstrates:

   a. acid mucosubstances
   b. the viability of the Schiff reagent
   c. sites where glycogen was removed
   d. areas of non-specific PAS-positive staining

4. Which of the following pigments is birefringent?

   a. formalin
   b. bile
   c. lipofuscin
   d. melanin

5. Acid mucosubstances and neutral mucosubstances can be differentiated by staining with both:

   a. mucicarmine and Weigert iron hematoxylin
   b. alcian blue and PAS
   c. toluidine blue and aldehyde fuchsin
   d. Sudan black and best carmine

6. In the colloidal iron method of staining, the principle of the reaction is believed to be the formation of an ionic bond between ferric iron and the free carboxyl group of:

   a. glycogen
   b. lipoproteins
   c. neutral mucins
   d. acid mucopolysaccharides

7. In order to suppress background and non-specific staining, a Congo red solution frequently contains:

   a. sodium acetate
   b. sodium chloride
   c. sodium phosphate
   d. sodium sulfate

8. In metachromatic staining, strong acid mucosubstances can be distinguished from weakly-acid mucosubstances by varying the:

   a. electrolyte concentration
   b. staining time
   c. temperature
   d. pH

9. The PAS reaction is useful for the demonstration of:

   a. hyaluronic acid
   b. dermatan sulfate
   c. chondroitin sulfate B
   d. neutral mucopolysaccharides

10. A section of muscle has been stained with the Verhoeff-van Gieson procedure. Microscopic examination shows blue-black nuclei, pale pink collagen, and unstained muscle fibers. The significance of these results is that the:

    a. section was overstained in iron hematoxylin
    b. staining in van Gieson solution was prolonged
    c. picric acid was too dilute
    d. stain results are as expected

11. A lymph node is stained with a silver method for reticulin and counterstained with nuclear fast red. After dehydration, there is a film over the entire slide that remains through clearing and coverslipping. The most likely cause is that the:

    a. unreacted silver remained on the slide
    b. nuclear fast red solution was too concentrated
    c. silver solution was contaminated by metal forceps
    d. slides were not rinsed with water after counterstaining

12. Yellow-brown pigment, often found in cardiac muscle and liver cells in increasing amounts with age or debilitated states, is known as:

    a. porphyrin
    b. hemoglobin
    c. lipofuscin
    d. melanin

13. Hemosiderin, hemoglobin, and bile pigment are classified as:

    a. endogenous pigments
    b. artifact pigments
    c. exogenous pigments
    d. extraneous pigments

14. The most appropriate hematoxylin solution for nuclear staining in a lengthy procedure that uses several very acidic solutions is one that is mordanted with:

    a. aluminum
    b. iron
    c. iodine
    d. tungsten

15. A modified phosphotungstic acid-hematoxylin procedure can be used to demonstrate:

    a. endothelial cells
    b. glial fibers
    c. Nissl substance
    d. Schwann cells

16. Which of the following is an argyrophil method?

    a. Fontana-Masson
    b. Gomori-Burtner
    c. Grimelius
    d. Weigert iron hematoxylin

17. In the Bodian technique, interference with primary staining may occur with prolonged treatment in:

    a. sodium thiosulfate
    b. oxalic acid
    c. gold chloride
    d. alcohol

18. The staining intensity of eosin is increased in muscle and red blood cells when tissues are fixed in:

    a. 10% neutral buffered formalin
    b. Zenker solution
    c. Carnoy solution
    d. Zamboni PAF solution

19. The laboratory has used all of the supply of aluminum hematoxylin solution. In order to prepare a new solution for immediate use, the solution must be:

a. prepared from hematein
b. air- and light-ripened
c. chemically oxidized
d. made in a small quantity

20. A commonly used connective tissue procedure that stains collagen blue is:

a. Masson trichrome
b. van Gieson
c. Movat pentachrome
d. aldehyde fuchsin

21. When using the cresyl echt violet method, Nissl substance and nuclei can be preferentially stained by varying the degree of differentiation and the:

a. alcohol concentration
b. dye concentration
c. staining time
d. solution pH

22. Muscle that histologically contains cytoplasmic cross-striations and has multiple nuclei located at the edge of the fibers is classified as:

a. smooth
b. visceral
c. skeletal
d. cardiac

23. A method for demonstrating nucleic acids in which DNA stains green and RNA stains red, is:

a. Feulgen reaction
b. methyl green-pyronin
c. Masson trichrome
d. Gomori trichrome

24. An effective counterstain following some silver impregnation procedures is:

a. acid fuchsin
b. aniline blue
c. picric acid
d. light green

25. The Fontana-Masson technique may be used to stain:

a. lipids
b. collagen
c. melanin
d. spirochetes

26. Which of the following is a regressive staining method for demonstrating a connective tissue component?

    a. Verhoeff-van Gieson
    b. Mallory aniline blue
    c. Masson trichrome
    d. Wilder reticulin

27. The differentiating solution in the Holzer method for glial fibers is:

    a. borax ferricyanide
    b. alcohol-acetone
    c. aniline oil-chloroform
    d. alcohol-dioxane

28. Which of the following staining procedures is preferred for demonstrating intracytoplasmic DNA-type viral inclusions in tissue?

    a. phloxine-methylene blue
    b. Feulgen
    c. PTAH
    d. Warthin-Starry

29. A solvent that is commonly used in oil red O and Sudan black B solutions to prevent the loss of lipids during fat staining is:

    a. xylene
    b. 70% ethanol
    c. acetone-ethanol
    d. propylene glycol

30. In the Verhoeff-van Gieson technique for demonstrating elastic fibers, the Verhoeff staining solution may be used for a few:

    a. hours
    b. days
    c. weeks
    d. months

31. A Ziehl-Neelsen procedure is done on a lung granuloma, but no acid-fast organisms are demonstrated. It would be wise to verify the absence of these organisms by using which of the following procedures?

    a. Grocott methenamine silver
    b. Truant auramine-rhodamine
    c. Warthin-Starry
    d. Gram

32. Microscopic inspection of a PAS-stained control section for fungi reveals very palely stained fungal organisms, making identification difficult. A likely cause for this problem is the:

    a. use of depleted Schiff reagent
    b. use of diluted chromic acid solution
    c. use of an incorrect reducing agent
    d. omission of sodium metabisulfite

33. A methyl green-pyronin procedure is done on a formalin-fixed section of tissue, but there is no evident RNA. Unless the procedure has been modified for formalin fixation, which of the following fixatives would have given more desirable results in this situation?

   a. Bouin
   b. Carnoy
   c. Zenker
   d. Zamboni

34. Examples of natural dyes are:

   a. hematoxylin, eosin, and methylene blue
   b. aniline blue, carmine, and hematoxylin
   c. crystal violet, methyl green, and indigo
   d. hematoxylin, carmine, and indigo

35. A chemical that will bleach melanin is:

   a. oxalic acid
   b. hydrogen peroxide
   c. sodium iodate
   d. sodium thiosulfate

36. Which of the following characteristics of ammoniacal silver solutions may cause tissue sections to wash off during impregnation?

   a. osmotic pressure
   b. alkalinity
   c. concentration
   d. temperature

37. The primary staining solution used in the Schmorl technique contains ferric chloride and potassium:

   a. dichromate
   b. iodide
   c. ferricyanide
   d. ferrocyanide

38. Which of the following procedures stains fibrin blue, nuclei blue, and collagen red?

   a. Gomori aldehyde fuchsin
   b. Mallory phosphotungstic acid-hematoxylin
   c. Gomori one-step trichrome
   d. periodic acid-Schiff-hematoxylin

39. In the Verhoeff-van Gieson technique for demonstrating elastic fibers, the Verhoeff staining solution is:

   a. made fresh before each use
   b. aged before use
   c. satisfactory for use indefinitely
   d. satisfactory for use up to one month

40. Microscopic review of a section stained with the Warthin-Starry technique shows the spirochetes stained yellow. The most likely cause of this problem is:

    a. overoxidizing
    b. underdeveloping
    c. use of impure reagents
    d. improper pH

41. Argentaffin cells found in the epithelium of the stomach and intestines are known as which of the following cells?

    a. amphophilic
    b. enterochromaffin
    c. absorptive
    d. Paneth

42. Which of the following substances is used in acid-fast staining procedures to enhance carbol-fuchsin staining and aid in dissolving the fuchsin dye?

    a. hydrochloric acid
    b. methylene blue
    c. phenol
    d. water

43. True epithelial cells lining ventricles and the spinal canal are called:

    a. astrocytes
    b. oligodendroglia
    c. microglia
    d. ependymal

44. Solutions of anionic dyes in picric acid are used to demonstrate:

    a. reticulin
    b. fibrocartilage
    c. collagen
    d. elastin

45. Which of the following pigments can be stained with Sudan black B and carbol fuchsin?

    a. bilirubin
    b. hemoglobin
    c. lipofuscin
    d. melanin

46. Transitional epithelium refers to:

    a. endothelium
    b. urothelium
    c. mesothelium
    d. metaplasia

47. Microscopic evaluation of a Brown & Brenn-stained control section shows the presence of gram-positive organisms, but no gram-negative organisms. This problem is most likely caused by:

a. reduced treatment with iodine
b. prolonged differentiation in Gallego solution
c. overdifferentiation in picric acid-acetone
d. decreased staining with crystal violet

48. Which of the following elastic stains perform well after any fixative, gives intense black staining of coarse fibers, must be differentiated microscopically, and gives permanent results with little fading?

a. PTAH
b. Verhoeff
c. Weigert
d. Masson

49. The addition of thymol crystals to staining solutions used for demonstrating microorganisms serves to:

a. maintain a neutral pH
b. facilitate reagent penetration
c. inhibit mold growth
d. help section adherence

50. A technique that can be used to demonstrate lipids in paraffin sections is:

a. staining with Sudan IV
b. fixation with osmium tetroxide
c. fixation with potassium dichromate
d. staining with alizarin red S

51. The reducing agent in diamine silver procedures for reticulin demonstration is most frequently:

a. formaldehyde
b. hydroquinone
c. pyridine
d. pyrogallol

52. The basic component of the central nervous system is the:

a. axon
b. neuron
c. dendrite
d. ganglion

53. Which of the following combination of stains will demonstrate both the myelin sheath and nerve fibers?

a. gallocyanine and Bodian
b. Nonidez and Bielschowsky
c. Luxol fast blue and Holmes
d. Sevier-Munger and thionin

54. A silver impregnation technique for demonstrating neurofibrils that uses formalin as a reducing agent is the ___ technique.

a. Hotchkiss-McManus
b. Pal-Weigert
c. Gros-Bielschowsky
d. Gomori-Burtner

55. The most consistently reliable technique for demonstrating fungi in tissues is the:

a. Gridley
b. Brown and Brenn
c. Grocott methenamine-silver
d. Ziehl-Neelsen

56. In addition to hematoxylin and potassium or ammonium alum, a traditional solution of Mayer hematoxylin contains:

a. 95% alcohol and glycerol
b. 95% alcohol, glycerol, and acetic acid
c. sodium iodate, chloral hydrate, and acetic acid
d. sodium iodate, chloral hydrate and citric acid

57. For light microscopic evaluation it is generally necessary to use special stains to demonstrate fungi in tissue sections because fungi:

a. can only be seen using silver impregnation
b. are removed in the routine staining process
c. stain variably with the H&E procedure
d. are never demonstrated with routine procedures

58. Which of the following staining procedures is most suitable for demonstrating general tissue morphology?

a. periodic acid-Schiff
b. Verhoeff-van Gieson
c. hematoxylin and eosin
d. Wilder reticulin

59. An example of an exogenous pigment is:

a. argentaffin
b. melanin
c. chromaffin
d. carbon

60. The sequence of reactions in the Wilder and Snook ammoniacal silver methods for demonstrating reticulin fibers is:

a. sensitization, oxidation, silver impregnation, reduction
b. oxidation, sensitization, silver impregnation, reduction
c. oxidation, sensitization, reduction, silver impregnation
d. sensitization, silver impregnation, oxidation, reduction

61. The Gomori ammoniacal silver technique for demonstrating reticulin will also demonstrate:

    a. small brain capillaries
    b. astrocytes
    c. nerve fibers
    d. myelin

62. The largest portion of the brain is the:

    a. medulla
    b. midbrain
    c. cerebellum
    d. cerebrum

63. Hemosiderin-laden macrophages present in the alveolar spaces of the lung can be distinguished from other pigmented macrophages by staining with:

    a. Prussian blue
    b. Fouchet reagent
    c. silver nitrate
    d. azocarmine B

64. The pigment commonly known as "wear and tear pigment" or "brown atrophy" is:

    a. hemofuchsin
    b. ceroid
    c. lipofuscin
    d. hemosiderin

65. To properly classify bone, it may be described as:

    a. glial and astrocytic
    b. cancellous and compact
    c. smooth and striated
    d. ground substance

66. Melanin is normally found in the:

    a. kidney
    b. liver
    c. skin
    d. stomach

67. A Gram stain has been done on a reactive, inflammatory lymph node, and the background structures are stained intense red, making identification of gram-negative organisms very difficult. This is most likely due to:

    a. prolonged staining with basic fuchsin
    b. drying following the crystal violet
    c. poor differentiation with picric acid-acetone
    d. incomplete dehydration and clearing

68. Which of the following acids in an alcoholic solution is most commonly used to differentiate aluminum-hematoxylin stained sections?

   a. formic
   b. hydrochloric
   c. sulfuric
   d. acetic

69. In the orcinol-new fuchsin technique, elastic fibers stain:

   a. blue-black to black
   b. red to reddish-brown
   c. blue to blue-green
   d. deep violet tinged with brown

70. Which of the following is a metachromatic stain used for identifying neurons and neuroglial cells?

   a. aniline blue
   b. Luxol fast blue
   c. toluidine blue
   d. Giemsa

71. Connective tissue proper refers to tissue composed of:

   a. spongy, cancellous, and cortical bone
   b. hyaline and fibrocartilage
   c. hematopoietic bone marrow
   d. collagen, reticulin, and elastin

72. A staining method used to demonstrate microglia is:

   a. Bielschowsky
   b. Luxol fast blue
   c. Del Rio-Hortega
   d. Cajal

73. The purpose of iodine in Gram procedures for staining bacteria is to:

   a. make the cell walls of bacteria permeable
   b. form a dye lake with crystal violet
   c. decolorize crystal violet
   d. inactivate bacteria

74. The terms "squamous", "cuboidal", and "columnar" describe cells that have their origin in which tissue?

   a. connective
   b. muscle
   c. epithelial
   d. bone

75. The atomic grouping within a dye that gives it its color is called a(n):

    a. auxochrome
    b. chromogen
    c. chromophore
    d. lake

76. In which of the following staining methods for nerve fibers is hydroquinone used?

    a. Mallory
    b. Weil
    c. Bodian
    d. Holzer

77. The reagent used for adjusting the pH to 3.4 in the Gomori trichrome stain solution for use on frozen sections of muscle is 1 N:

    a. HCl
    b. NH_4OH
    c. HNO_3
    d. NaOH

78. The purpose of classifying bacteria as either gram-positive or gram-negative is to:

    a. differentiate between cocci and bacilli
    b. determine susceptibility of organisms for certain treatment
    c. eliminate the need for specific cultures of organisms
    d. allow definitive identification for *M. tuberculosis*

79. Which of the following chemicals is used as both a mordant and a differentiator in the Heidenhain hematoxylin procedure for demonstrating amebae?

    a. mercuric chloride
    b. chromium aluminum sulfate
    c. aluminum ammonium sulfate
    d. ferric ammonium sulfate

80. Fixation of tissues for 2 weeks in which of the following will most likely impair nuclear staining?

    a. neutral buffered formalin
    b. Zenker solution
    c. paraformaldehyde
    d. glyoxal

81. A researcher wishes to differentiate the different types of granulocytes in a tissue section. The stain of choice is a_____ stain.

    a. Gram
    b. acid-fast
    c. Romanowsky
    d. silver impregnation

82. A substance that has the ability to both bind silver and reduce it to a visible metallic form is said to be:

    a. argyrophilic
    b. argentaffin
    c. amphophilic
    d. auxochromic

83. After H&E staining, the cytoplasm in a tissue section appears hazy, obscure, and contrasts poorly with the nuclei. The most likely cause is that:

    a. eosin Y was used
    b. phloxine was added to the eosin
    c. acetic acid was present in the eosin solution
    d. slides were not differentiated properly in alcohol

84. Rinsing in alcohol or water after primary stain application should be avoided in the thionin method for demonstrating Nissl substance because:

    a. sections will be overstained
    b. an undesirable precipitate will form
    c. the primary stain will be removed
    d. the Nissl substance will be dissolved

85. Microscopic review of auramine-rhodamine stained control slides will reveal:

    a. fungal organisms
    b. yeast forms
    c. mycobacteria
    d. spirochetes

86. A dye in which the coloring elements are found in the anionic portion of the compound is a(n):

    a. acid dye
    b. basic dye
    c. amphoteric dye
    d. polychromatic dye

87. The Stein and Hall techniques are based on the conversion of bile pigment to:

    a. porphyrins
    b. biliverdin
    c. hemoglobin
    d. aposiderin

88. The acid used in the Prussian blue reaction is:

    a. acetic
    b. hydrochloric
    c. nitric
    d. sulfuric

89. Areolar connective tissue is also known as:

    a. mineralized connective tissue
    b. dense connective tissue
    c. loose connective tissue
    d. specialized connective tissue

90. A hematoxylin solution that is only used progressively is:

    a. Harris
    b. Ehrlich
    c. Mayer
    d. Delafield

91. Nuclei stained with a new Harris hematoxylin solution are predominately red and imprecisely outlined. This is most likely because of the use of:

    a. insufficient differentiation
    b. prolonged neutralization
    c. incompletely oxidized hematoxylin
    d. a non-acidified hematoxylin solution

92. In the Hall method, Fouchet reagent is used to demonstrate:

    a. copper
    b. bile
    c. lipofuscin
    d. melanin

93. To achieve the desired intensity of purple when using the Gomori aldehyde fuchsin stain for demonstrating elastic tissue, the paraldehyde used to prepare the reagent should be:

    a. aged
    b. fresh
    c. chilled
    d. heated

94. Microscopic examination of an H&E-stained section shows a pink artifact surrounding the tissue and in tissue spaces. The most probable cause of this artifact is:

    a. precipitation of the eosin
    b. excess acetic acid in the eosin
    c. surplus adhesive on the slide
    d. poor bluing of the hematoxylin

95. In the Mallory phosphotungstic acid-hematoxylin (PTAH) method, skeletal muscle striations stain:

    a. blue
    b. red
    c. black
    d. yellow

96. Acidophilic tissue components that should appear stained different shades of pink following H&E staining are:

    a. muscle, collagen, and erythrocytes
    b. muscle, reticulin, and elastin
    c. collagen, basement membrane, and nucleic acids

97. In order for the Gram stain to work properly, it is important to apply the mordant:

    a. after the crystal violet
    b. prior to any of the stains
    c. combined with the primary dye
    d. after the counterstain

98. Which of the following methods use a methenamine solution?

    a. Foot-Bielschowsky and Bodian
    b. Wilder and Snook
    c. Jones and Gomori
    d. Gridley and Laidlaw

99. The purpose of an acetic acid rinse in the Gomori one-step trichrome procedure is to:

    a. differentiate the nuclear staining
    b. make color shades more transparent
    c. permit tungstate ions to bind to collagen
    d. facilitate muscle staining with chromotrope 2R

100. Differential staining of nuclei and cytoplasm with Giemsa solution is an example of:

    a. polychromasia
    b. metachromasia
    c. orthochromasia
    d. hypochromasia

101. Which of the following histological features is unique to cardiac muscle?

    a. cross-striations
    b. peripherally located nuclei
    c. intercalated discs
    d. non-branching fibers

102. Pigment that is present on the surface of cells but not within them is probably:

    a. endogenous
    b. hematogenous
    c. hepatogenous
    d. artifactual

103. Oligodendroglia are cells that function in the production and maintenance of myelin sheaths that surround:

    a. axons
    b. neuroglia
    c. microglia
    d. astrocytes

104. Which of the following is an example of a metachromatic stain?

    a. Congo red
    b. orange G
    c. toluidine blue
    d. thioflavin T

105. Hemosiderin can be removed from tissue by treating the sections with a dilute solution of:

    a. Lugol iodine
    b. hydrogen peroxide
    c. sulfuric acid
    d. alcoholic ammonium hydroxide

106. Which of the following procedures will demonstrate most amoebae in tissue sections?

    a. Grocott methenamine-silver
    b. Kinyoun acid-fast
    c. Mayer mucicarmine
    d. periodic acid-Schiff

107. Which of the following is an iron hematoxylin solution that is frequently used for nuclear staining?

    a. Harris
    b. Delafield
    c. Mayer
    d. Weigert

108. The pigment that is formed following a reaction of ferrous ions with potassium ferricyanide is known as:

    a. Prussian blue
    b. methylene blue
    c. Turnbull blue
    d. Nile blue

109. Microscopic examination of a skeletal muscle section stained with PTAH reveals very pale pink staining of the collagen. The most common cause of this pale staining is:

    a. too concentrated a solution of oxalic acid
    b. overoxidized phosphotungstic acid hematoxylin
    c. prolonged water and alcohol rinses
    d. failure to postmordant in Zenker fluid

110. A staining procedure that allows correlative studies of cellular elements, fiber pathways, and vascular components of the nervous system is the Luxol fast blue combined with the____ stain.

    a. oil red O
    b. Holmes silver nitrate
    c. periodic acid-Schiff-hematoxylin
    d. cresyl fast violet

111. Cells that are numerous in connective tissue and have cytoplasmic granules that stain metachromatically are:

    a. Purkinje cells
    b. macrophages
    c. enterochromaffin cells
    d. mast cells

112. An elastic tissue stain that may also be useful for staining beta cells of pancreatic islets is:

    a. orcinol-new fuchsin
    b. Weigert resorcin-fuchsin
    c. Verhoeff-van Gieson
    d. Gomori aldehyde fuchsin

113. Stains for simple lipids are performed on which of the following sections:

    a. paraffin
    b. frozen
    c. celloidin
    d. glycol methacrylate

114. The toughest of the connective tissue fibers is:

    a. reticulin
    b. elastin
    c. collagen
    d. myelin

115. Which of the following is the only hematogenous pigment found in normal red blood cells?

    a. hemoglobin
    b. hemosiderin
    c. hematoidin
    d. hemozoon

116. Oil red O staining is based on the principle of:

    a. impregnation
    b. birefringence
    c. ionic linkages
    d. absorption

117. Which of the following methods involves the reduction of ferric ions to ferrous ions followed by precipitation with the Turnbull blue reaction?

a. Schmorl
b. Grimelius
c. Sevier-Munger
d. Gmelin

118. In the Gomori aldehyde fuchsin technique, elastic fibers stain:

a. blue to black
b. violet-purple
c. reddish-brown
d. bluish-green

119. In the Gomori technique, sodium urate crystals are stained with:

a. rubeanic acid
b. leucofuchsin
c. methenamine-silver
d. aldehyde fuchsin

120. A method that will selectively stain astrocytes in frozen sections is the:

a. Cajal gold sublimate
b. Sevier-Munger
c. Pal-Weigert
d. Mallory PTAH

121. Which of the following is an argyrophil stain for neurofibrils that can also be used to demonstrate neurosecretory granules?

a. Cajal
b. Fontana-Masson
c. Sevier-Munger
d. Weil

122. Some argentaffin cells are also known as:

a. Kupffer cells
b. Grimelius cells
c. Paneth cells
d. Kulchitsky cells

123. Which of the following acts as the differentiating solution in the Verhoeff-van Gieson procedure?

a. Weigert iodine solution
b. borax ferricyanide
c. ferric chloride
d. acid alcohol

124. The staining mechanism in which metallic substances are selectively deposited on structures and made visible by reduction of the metal is called:

    a. substantive
    b. adjective
    c. progressive
    d. impregnation

125. *Entamoeba histolytica* can be demonstrated well with which of the following procedures or methods?

    a. Gordon-Sweets
    b. von Kossa
    c. periodic acid-Schiff
    d. Schmorl

126. In the Gomori one-step trichrome stain, collagen stains:

    a. yellow
    b. green
    c. black
    d. red

127. In humans, nonkeratinizing stratified squamous epithelium is found covering/lining the:

    a. skin
    b. trachea
    c. esophagus
    d. urinary bladder

128. The cytoplasmic granules in connective tissue mast cells stain well with:

    a. toluidine blue
    b. eosin
    c. phloxine
    d. orange G

129. Granules found in cells of the adrenal medulla that appear brown when fixed in Orth solution are called:

    a. melanin
    b. lipofuscin
    c. chromaffin
    d. chromatin

130. In the Weigert stain for fibrin, the principal coloring agent is:

    a. periodic acid
    b. crystal violet
    c. Ponceau-fuchsin
    d. phosphotungstic acid-hematoxylin

131. Microscopic examination of an H&E-stained brain section reveals basophilic material in the cytoplasm of the neurons. This material is most likely:

   a. secretory granules
   b. neurofilaments
   c. RNA
   d. lipids

132. Which of the following methods is a modification of the Bodian technique that uses a buffered impregnating solution to increase the specificity of the stain?

   a. Rio-Hortega
   b. Nonidez
   c. Bielschowsky
   d. Holmes

133. Which of the following stains is dependent upon differences in the bacterial cell wall for differential staining?

   a. Gridley
   b. Gram
   c. Grocott
   d. Warthin-Starry

134. Acid-alcohol decolorizers are generally recommended over aqueous decolorizers for use with acid-fast procedures because alcoholic solutions:

   a. are more stable
   b. begin dehydration
   c. penetrate more slowly
   d. allow more uniform decolorization

135. A section of which of the following provides a control when demonstrating elastic fibers?

   a. lung
   b. kidney
   c. spleen
   d. liver

136. Which of the following hematoxylin solutions contains ethylene glycol and aluminum sulfate?

   a. Harris
   b. Delafield
   c. Gill
   d. Mayer

137. A tumor or new growth largely made up of nerve cells is called a(n):

   a. osteoma
   b. neuroma
   c. lipoma
   d. fibroma

138. In the Jones and Gomori methenamine-silver techniques for basement membranes, sections are oxidized with:

    a. potassium permanganate
    b. chromic acid
    c. lithium carbonate
    d. periodic acid

139. To aid in the specific identification of a mycotic infection, which of the following techniques may be used?

    a. Schmorl
    b. fluorescent antibody (FA)
    c. MacCallum-Goodpasture
    d. Sevier-Munger

140. A component of nerve tissue that can be demonstrated by gold and silver impregnation techniques is/are:

    a. neurofibrils
    b. Nissl substance
    c. Schwann cells
    d. myelin

141. Nissl substance can be demonstrated with which of the following stains?

    a. thionin and cresyl echt violet
    b. eosin and phloxine
    c. silver nitrate and gold sublimate
    d. orange G and methyl blue

142. Tissue intended for Brown-Hopps staining of gram-positive and gram-negative bacteria is fixed in Bouin solution. The most likely effect of this fixative on staining results is to:

    a. enhance staining
    b. inhibit staining
    c. have no effect on staining
    d. completely eliminate staining

143. In the Wilder technique for demonstrating reticulin, uranyl nitrate acts as a(n):

    a. mordant
    b. accentuator
    c. sensitizer
    d. toner

144. Microscopic evaluation of an H&E-stained section reveals dark deposits of material dispersed irregularly over the tissue. The most likely cause of this problem is that the hematoxylin solution:

    a. was not filtered before use
    b. is past its useful shelf life
    c. contains too much acetic acid
    d. does not contain an oxidizer

145. Microscopic review of a GMS-stained section shows elastic fibers, crenated red cells, and mucin all stained black. This is most likely the result of:

a. overexposure to hot methenamine silver
b. underexposure to gold chloride
c. underexposure to sodium thiosulfate
d. performing the procedure in a microwave oven

146. During microscopic examination of a fungus stain, extraneous fungal elements are seen above rather than in the section. The most likely cause for this problem is:

a. poor dehydration prior to coverslipping
b. prolonged exposure to silver solution
c. contaminated staining solutions
d. a bacterial rather than fungal disease

147. Sections of lung stained with GMS and PAS show positive staining of what appear to be crypto-coccal organisms. However, the same oval-shaped bodies are seen in non-granulomatous areas and on edges of the tissue. This "positive" staining material is therefore most likely:

a. calcium
b. ceroid
c. talcum powder
d. asbestos

148. Spirochetes are filamentous bacteria that are known to be:

a. argentophilic
b. argyrophilic
c. polychromatic
d. metachromatic

149. Following hematoxylin and eosin staining, slides are dehydrated through ascending strengths of alcohol and cleared in xylene; however, the first xylene in the series is milky white. The most appropriate action is to:

a. change all solutions in the staining series
b. change xylenes at the end of the series
c. change alcohols and xylenes at the end of the series
d. air-dry slides and dehydrateand clear as usual

150. In the Warthin-Starry technique, occasional staining of nuclei, melanin, and other pigments may interfere with identification of the microorganisms. Modifications in the staining procedure that might eliminate this problem are:

a. prolonged development and a lower pH
b. prolonged development and a higher pH
c. shorter development and a lower pH
d. shorter development and a higher pH

151. If hematoxylin is unavailable, which of the following dyes is recommended as a substitute in a routine hematoxylin and eosin procedure?

   a. methyl blue
   b. aniline blue
   c. Nile blue A
   d. celestine blue

152. The phosphotungstic acid-hematoxylin (PTAH) stain is useful for demonstrating:

   a. edema fluid
   b. muscle striations
   c. ground substance
   d. reticulin network

153. Hemosiderin is thought to be composed of ferric iron and:

   a. protein
   b. collagen
   c. chromatin
   d. fatty acids

154. The density of collagen fibers in any given organ varies from "loose" to "dense" according to the:

   a. heredity and sex of the individual
   b. location and function
   c. size of the organ
   d. age of the individual

155. In slides stained with hematoxylin and eosin, the sections appear very pink, with pale-reddish brown nuclei. Of the following, the most appropriate action is to:

   a. restain the sections for a longer time in hematoxylin
   b. discard and replace the ammonia water
   c. replace the hematoxylin with fresh solution
   d. change all solutions and restain sections

156. In silver impregnation techniques, the use of improperly cleaned glassware results in:

   a. the absence of silver staining
   b. nonselective silver precipitation
   c. inadequate counterstaining
   d. the inability to tone

157. Which of the following methods stains elastic tissue brown?

   a. acid orcein
   b. resorcin-fuchsin
   c. Gomori aldehyde fuchsin
   d. Verhoeff-van Gieson

158. The function of potassium permanganate in the phosphotungstic acid-hematoxylin (PTAH) method is thought to be that of a:

a. sensitizer
b. mordant
c. differentiator
d. dye-trapping agent

159. A hematoxylin stain primarily used to demonstrate amoebae is:

a. Harris aluminum
b. Heidenhain iron
c. Pal-Weigert iron
d. Mallory phosphotungstic acid

160. The pathologist has requested a Feulgen procedure on a lymph node. The staining sequence for this procedure is:

a. hydrochloric acid, sulfurous acid, Schiff, light green
b. periodic acid, Schiff, sulfurous acid, light green
c. hydrochloric acid, Schiff, sulfurous acid, light green
d. Schiff, hydrochloric acid, light green

161. Fresh silver solutions were properly prepared and used in a Warthin-Starry technique. After completion of the procedure, the positive control does not demonstrate spirochetes. Of the following, the most likely reason for this problem is:

a. poorly fixed tissue
b. contaminated glassware
c. improperly prepared reducing solution
d. incorrectly selected mordant

162. The function of Bouin fluid in trichrome stains is that of a(n):

a. mordant
b. reducer
c. oxidizer
d. sensitizer

163. In order to protect the leprosy organism from extraction of the acid-fast component, sections are deparaffinized in xylene and:

a. peanut oil
b. dioxane
c. alcohol
d. acetone

164. In the Verhoeff-van Gieson technique, ferric chloride and iodine in the Verhoeff solution function initially as mordants and then as:

a. neutralizers
b. differentiators
c. sensitizers
d. oxidizers

165. A black pigment that is insoluble, often found in the lungs and hilar lymph nodes, cannot be bleached, and cannot be identified by typical chemical reactions for pigments is most likely:

a. hemosiderin
b. melanin
c. lipofuscin
d. anthracotic

166. Which of the following tissue components can be stained by Weigert resorcin-fuchsin, Hart resorcin-fuchsin, or orcinol-new fuchsin?

a. reticular fibers
b. myosin fibers
c. elastic fibers
d. collagen fibers

167. Sections stained with the Grocott procedure for fungi were originally completely satisfactory. After several weeks of being exposed to light, however, a granular black precipitate can be seen over the sections. This is most likely due to the omission during staining of:

a. chromic acid
b. gold chloride
c. sodium bisulfite
d. sodium thiosulfate

168. The routine staining procedures for liver biopsies include duplicate H&E, PAS with and without diastase, trichrome, reticulin, and iron stains. While doing the stains, a trichrome stain is accidentally done on the slide designated for PAS without diastase. There are no more unstained sections. Aside from cutting more sections, which of the following stained sections would be best to destain and then stain for PAS without diastase?

a. trichrome
b. PAS with diastase
c. reticulin
d. H&E

169. Mordants are generally classified as:

a. amphoteric
b. weakly acidic
c. metallic
d. gaseous

170. The oxidizer in the Gridley procedure for reticulin fibers is:

a. potassium permanganate
b. phosphomolybdic acid
c. periodic acid
d. chromic acid

171. A rapid bile identification technique that involves destruction of tissue sections by acid is the:

a. Gmelin test
b. Ralph method
c. Hall technique
d. Gomori reaction

172. The oxidizer used in the Gomori reticulin method is:

a. periodic acid
b. chromic acid
c. potassium permanganate
d. phosphomolybdic acid

173. The purpose of nonmetallic forceps, acid-cleaned glassware, and triple-distilled water in silver techniques is to prevent:

a. premature uptake of silver
b. changes in pH of the silver solution
c. false-negative staining
d. contamination of the silver solution

174. Another name for fat cells is:

a. APUD cells
b. myocytes
c. adipocytes
d. histiocytes

175. Elastic fibers have an affinity for which of the following stains?

a. Sudan
b. indigo
c. brazilin
d. orcein

176. Of the following, the most reliable stain for demonstrating gram-negative bacteria in tissue sections is the:

a. Giemsa
b. Brown-Hopps
c. Ziehl-Neelsen
d. Grocott

177. A delicate 3-dimensional connective tissue meshwork that forms the framework of organs such as the spleen and lymph nodes is made of:

a. elastic fibers
b. reticular fibers
c. smooth muscle
d. basement membrane

178. Carmine and aluminum chloride combine to form Mayer:

    a. mucihematein
    b. alcoholic carmine
    c. carmalum
    d. mucicarmine

179. In the Bodian technique, Protargol™ impregnates both neurofibrils and connective tissue. Subsequently, connective tissue is rendered colorless by replacement of the silver with:

    a. copper
    b. gold
    c. lead
    d. tin

180. Cartilage is characterized by a solid intercellular substance that stains metachromatically called:

    a. chondromucin
    b. sarcoplasm
    c. ptyalin
    d. lacunae

181. The primary dye used in a rapid, non-silver staining procedure to demonstrate *Helicobacter pylori* is a/an:

    a. azure-eosin
    b. leucofuchsin
    c. colloidal iron
    d. carbol-fuchsin

182. The chromic acid-Schiff procedure that demonstrates the cell walls of fungi is known as the:

    a. Bauer method
    b. Levaditi method
    c. Baker method
    d. Schmorl method

183. A method that will stain hemoglobin emerald-green is:

    a. Gomori
    b. Dunn-Thompson
    c. Okajima
    d. Bauer

184. In the Feulgen reaction for nucleic acids, slides are placed in 1N hydrochloric acid to promote:

    a. autolysis
    b. oxidation
    c. hydrolysis
    d. anabolism

185. The Grocott methenamine-silver method can be used to demonstrate:

    a. uric acid
    b. argyrophilic cells
    c. hemosiderin
    d. copper

186. Important factors affecting gram-positive staining of some organisms include the:

    a. age of organisms and acidity of environment
    b. size of organisms and presence of lipid capsule
    c. shape and size of organisms
    d. time in crystal violet and safranin solutions

187. The Schmorl method will stain reducing substances:

    a. blue
    b. red
    c. black
    d. brown

188. Microscopic evaluation of a Wright-stained smear reveals poor nuclear staining and very little cytoplasmic differentiation. This is most likely the result of:

    a. an improper pH
    b. smears that are too thin
    c. the staining solution that is not ripened
    d. staining done at room temperature

189. A component in the cell nucleus that stains strongly with basic dyes is called:

    a. endoplasmic reticulum
    b. cytomembrane
    c. lipofuscin
    d. chromatin

190. The nerve process that carries electrical impulses away from the cell body is called a(n):

    a. neuron
    b. dendrite
    c. synapse
    d. axon

191. Differentiating agents in the Luxol fast blue procedure for myelin are:

    a. sodium borate and potassium ferrocyanide
    b. absolute alcohol and aniline oil
    c. gold chloride and sodium thiosulfate
    d. lithium carbonate and 70% alcohol

192. In the Masson trichrome method, muscle fibers are colored:

   a. red
   b. blue
   c. yellow
   d. green

193. The staining method considered to be most sensitive and specific for copper is the _____ method.

   a. chloranilic acid
   b. rhodanine
   c. orcein
   d. aldehyde fuchsin

194. The Mallory technique uses aniline blue to stain:

   a. reticulin
   b. muscle
   c. elastin
   d. collagen

195. Which of the following chemicals functions as an oxidizer?

   a. aluminum sulfate
   b. sodium sulfite
   c. potassium permanganate
   d. acetic acid

196. The most commonly used dye solution for staining *Mycobacterium tuberculosis* is composed of:

   a. basic fuchsin and phenol
   b. acid fuchsin and formalin
   c. acid fuchsin and carbolic acid
   d. new fuchsin and hydrochloric acid

197. Ammonia water, lithium carbonate solution, and Scott tap water substitute are examples of:

   a. decolorizers
   b. accentuators
   c. differentiators
   d. bluing agents

198. Procedures that demonstrate argentaffin granules include which of the following?

   a. Grimelius and Sevier-Munger
   b. Churukian-Schenck and Bodian
   c. Fontana-Masson and Gomori-Burtner
   d. Pascual and Gros-Schultze

199. An organism that is resistant to decolorization after staining with a basic aniline dye followed by an iodine mordant is referred to as:

a. acid-fast
b. argentaffin
c. gram-positive
d. argyrophilic

200. In the Brown-Hopps stain, one of the differentiating solutions is:

a. acid alcohol
b. Gram iodine
c. Gallego solution
d. 75% alcohol

201. In the Verhoeff-van Gieson technique, elastic fibers stain:

a. red to purple
b. blue-black to black
c. yellow to brown
d. blue to blue-green

202. The most commonly used phenolic compound for reducing adsorbed silver to a visible metallic state in argyrophil procedures such as the Warthin-Starry is:

a. sodium thiosulfate
b. uranyl nitrate
c. hydroquinone
d. sodium bisulfate

203. The term "argentaffin" literally denotes a reaction wherein cells have the ability to reduce a salt of:

a. chromium
b. lithium
c. copper
d. silver

204. When excessive melanin deposition interferes with examination of cellular morphology, melanin pigment can be removed by bleaching a section with:

a. sodium thiosulfate
b. hydroquinone
c. potassium permanganate
d. ammoniacal silver

205. The selectivity for nuclear staining by Harris hematoxylin can be increased by adding:

a. aluminum salts
b. sodium iodate
c. glycerol
d. alcohol

206. A stained section mounted with a synthetic resin appears cloudy. This is most likely the result of using a mounting medium that has:

a. a refractive index equal to that of the tissue
b. become too thick
c. been thinned too much with xylene
d. been applied to a dry slide

207. Thionin will stain Nissl substances because Nissl substance is:

a. argyrophilic
b. acidophilic
c. metachromatic
d. amphoteric

208. Filamentous structures known as "hyphae" are associated with which of the following microorganisms?

a. bacteria
b. protozoa
c. viruses
d. fungi

209. Picric acid, eosin, and tartrazine are examples of what type of dye?

a. basic
b. plasma
c. natural
d. fluorescent

210. Tissue composed of a network of bony trabeculae separated by interconnecting bone marrow spaces is characteristic of:

a. cortical bone
b. woven bone
c. compact bone
d. cancellous bone

211. Which of the following is the oxidizer in the Snook and Laidlaw methods for demonstrating reticulin fibers?

a. periodic acid
b. phosphomolybdic acid
c. ferric ammonium sulfate
d. potassium permanganate

212. The second differentiating solution used in the Weil method contains sodium borate and:

a. potassium ferrocyanide
b. potassium ferricyanide
c. ferric chloride
d. ferrous sulfate

213. The property of "acid-fastness" appears to be related to the walls of organisms that contain:

   a. lipid
   b. protein
   c. amyloid
   d. iron

214. A method sometimes used for increasing the diffusion rate of dye molecules and thereby increasing the rate of staining is by increasing the _____ of the dye solution.

   a. temperature
   b. osmolality
   c. alkalinity
   d. polychromasia

215. Which of the following connective tissue components is sudanophilic?

   a. elastin
   b. reticulin
   c. adipose
   d. cartilage

216. Which of the following groups of dyes are generally used for counterstaining?

   a. metanil yellow, methylene blue, Prussian blue
   b. methylene blue, methyl green, nuclear fast red
   c. eosin, phloxine, carmine
   d. eosin, metanil yellow, orcein

217. A technique for demonstrating calcium wherein sections immersed in silver nitrate solution are exposed to bright light is the:

   a. Schmorl
   b. von Kossa
   c. dopa oxidase
   d. alizarin red S

218. In the Holzer method, glial fibers are stained with:

   a. silver nitrate
   b. crystal violet
   c. orcein
   d. Protargol™

219. Commonly used mordants for making hematoxylin solutions are:

   a. ammonium aluminum sulfate and ferric ammonium sulfate
   b. potassium aluminum sulfate and potassium permanganate
   c. phosphotungstic acid and phosphomolybdic acid
   d. potassium permanganate and ferric chloride

220. Microscopic examination of a bone marrow aspirate smear stained with Giemsa shows blue-gray erythrocytes and blue leukocytes. The most likely explanation for this result is that the:

   a. cells are staining correctly for this procedure
   b. staining solution is too alkaline
   c. staining solution is too acid
   d. smear is from an anemic patient

221. Tissues from which of the following organs provide the best control for reticulin stains?

   a. heart
   b. uterus
   c. liver
   d. lung

222. In the Masson trichrome procedure, after staining with Biebrich scarlet-acid fuchsin, sections are differentiated with:

   a. 1% hydrochloric acid in 70% alcohol
   b. dilute aqueous solution of acetic acid
   c. phosphomolybdic-phosphotungstic acid
   d. dilute ferric ammonium sulfate

223. Which of the following is an example of a basic dye?

   a. toluidine blue
   b. ponceau S
   c. orange G
   d. acridine orange

224. Nissl substance is predominantly composed of:

   a. collagenous fibers
   b. neurofibrillary tangles
   c. rough endoplasmic reticulum
   d. microsomes and microtubules

225. Two controls may be necessary to check the strength of a phosphotungstic acid-hematoxylin solution, depending on the purpose of the stain. The correct control pair is striated muscle and:

   a. liver
   b. spleen
   c. ovary
   d. brain

226. Aldehyde fuchsin to be used for elastic stains is generally stable for:

   a. one week at room temperature
   b. 3 to 4 weeks at 4°C
   c. up to a year at 4°C
   d. indefinitely

227. A combination method for demonstrating fat and myelin in frozen sections of brain is the Luxol fast blue stain combined with:

a. PAS
b. oil red O
c. H&E
d. PTAH

228. A possible cause of poor staining by Gomori aldehyde fuchsin solution is that:

a. fresh paraldehyde was used
b. the dye was not the correct color index
c. hydrochloric acid was used
d. 70% ethanol was used as the dye solvent

229. Argentaffin procedures can be made more specific for melanin by first oxidizing non-melanin reducing substances using:

a. sodium thiosulfate
b. ammoniacal silver
c. hydroquinone
d. iodine

230. The bacterium *Legionella pneumophila* can be demonstrated using which staining method?

a. Schleifstein
b. Pinkerton
c. May-Grunwald
d. Steiner

231. Some dye solutions are made colorless by reduction, used for identification of specific tissue components, and then reoxidized to restore the color. The term applied to these colorless compounds is:

a. xanthanes
b. chromophoric
c. leuco
d. peroxidases

232. In neurons, chromatolysis refers to the loss of:

a. axons
b. Nissl substance
c. dendrites
d. myelin

233. Because melanin can bind and reduce silver without the use of a separate reducing agent, it is said to be:

a. argentaffin
b. amphoteric
c. argyrophilic
d. achromatic

234. In silver impregnation methods, gold chloride is used as a(n):

    a. sensitizer
    b. reducer
    c. toner
    d. oxidizer

235. A staining method for distinguishing muscle, elastic fibers, and collagen/reticular fibers from one another is:

    a. Movat pentachrome
    b. Mallory aniline blue
    c. Lillie allochrome
    d. Mallory PTAH

236. In the Hotchkiss-McManus PAS technique, polysaccharides present in fungal walls are oxidized by:

    a. potassium permanganate
    b. periodic acid
    c. phosphotungstic acid
    d. chromic acid

237. The connective tissue cells actively involved in wound repair are:

    a. plasma cells
    b. mast cells
    c. adipocytes
    d. fibroblasts

238. The most appropriate method for demonstrating acid-fast organisms that are difficult to stain by other methods is the _____ method.

    a. Ziehl-Neelsen
    b. Gridley
    c. Kinyoun
    d. Wade

239. In acid-fast staining, drying of the section after carbol-fuchsin staining should be avoided because repeated attempts at removing the insoluble compound formed by drying may result in:

    a. complete decolorization of organisms
    b. an opaque background
    c. "beaded" red organisms
    d. poor counterstaining

240. The process by which the mineral content of tissues can be studied following removal of organic tissue components is called:

   a. microincineration
   b. enzyme histochemistry
   c. in-situ hybridization
   d. autoradiography

241. Insoluble compounds that resist decolorization with ether-acetone are noted on microscopic evaluation of a control section stained with the Brown-Hopps stain. The presence of these compounds is probably due to:

   a. inadequate fixation
   b. inadequate dehydration
   c. omission of mordant during staining
   d. sections being allowed to dry during staining

242. In staining methods for demonstrating reticulin, potassium permanganate, phosphomolybdic acid, and periodic acid function as:

   a. reducers
   b. oxidizers
   c. sensitizers
   d. toners

243. To demonstrate degenerating myelin, the Marchi method uses:

   a. osmium tetroxide
   b. oil red O
   c. silver nitrate
   d. crystal violet

244. A phosphotungstic acid-hematoxylin solution can be ripened for immediate use by adding:

   a. potassium permanganate
   b. aluminum sulfate
   c. acetic acid
   d. alcohol

245. The staining of simple fats with lipid-soluble dyes depends on:

   a. Van der Waals forces
   b. physical processes
   c. hydrogen bonds
   d. Brownian motion

246. Two eosinophilic tissue components that may be difficult to distinguish morphologically are:

   a. elastic and skeletal muscle
   b. cartilage and ground substance
   c. collagen and smooth muscle
   d. peripheral nerve and cardiac muscle

247. Small amounts of ferric iron are normally found in the:

a. liver
b. lung
c. spleen
d. kidney

248. Which of the following methods uses ammoniacal silver carbonate for impregnation of neurofibrils?

a. Rio-Hortega
b. Nonidez
c. Holzer
d. Marchi

249. Sections are stained with Harris hematoxylin for 5 minutes and then treated with dilute hydrochloric acid. This type of staining is referred to as:

a. impregnation
b. progressive
c. regressive
d. absorption

250. The color range seen in Romanowsky stains is the result of:

a. methyl green and orange G
b. the use of pure methylene blue
c. a combination of pthalocyanine and nitro dyes
d. the combination of derivatives of methylene blue with eosin

251. The major disadvantage of using the crystal violet technique for the demonstration of amyloid is that:

a. only alpha amyloid can be demonstrated
b. it requires a polarizing microscope for verification
c. amyloid does not contrast with connective tissue
d. the preparation is not permanent

252. A tissue has been fixed in neutral-buffered formalin. To achieve optimum results with the Mallory PTAH stain, the microscopic sections should be:

a. cut at 10 micrometers
b. stained with freshly prepared solution
c. mordanted in Bouin fixative
d. mordanted in Zenker fixative

253. When checking a control slide stained with Luxol fast blue, a good stain should show a sharp differentiation between:

a. astrocytes and microglia
b. Nissl substance and nuclei
c. gray and white matter
d. glial fibers and axons

254. Colophonium (rosin) is used in the Wohlbach-Giemsa technique to:

a. lower the pH of the staining solution
b. mordant the stain
c. act as a sensitizer on the tissue
d. differentiate the tissue elements

255. A PTAH staining solution produces the best results when it is:

a. prepared fresh
b. heated to 38°C for staining
c. oxidized with ferric chloride
d. allowed to oxidize naturally

256. *Mycobacterium tuberculosis* may be demonstrated with which of the following stains?

a. crystal violet
b. leucofuchsin
c. acid fuchsin
d. carbol-fuchsin

257. Which of the following is a hydrophobic mounting medium?

a. synthetic resin
b. gelatin
c. glycerol
d. gum syrup

258. Spirochetes in fixed tissue are best demonstrated by:

a. enzyme histochemistry
b. vital staining
c. metallic impregnation
d. physical methods

259. Sections stained with oil-soluble dyes must be mounted in a medium which:

a. is dissolved in a hydrocarbon
b. has a high refractive index
c. will retain lipids
d. is permanent

260. Fite, Ziehl-Neelsen, and Kinyoun are names associated with:

a. microfilaments
b. microorganisms
c. microvilli
d. microtubules

261. In the Feulgen reaction, hydrochloric acid reacts with DNA to create:

a. polynucleotides
b. base pairs
c. methyl groups
d. aldehyde groups

262. Tissue from which of the following organs should be selected as a control for the alcian blue technique (pH 2.5)?

a. skin
b. kidney
c. muscle
d. colon

263. The silver nitrate technique of Fontana may be used to demonstrate:

a. spirochete organisms
b. calcium deposits
c. elastic fibers
d. argentaffin cells

264. Sections were stained using the microwave oven. The tissue at the top of the slide stained darker than that at the bottom portion. To prevent this from happening in the future:

a. increase oven wattage and be sure to maintain exposure times
b. increase exposure times and be sure to maintain wattage
c. place the slides toward the back of the oven
d. remove slides from the oven and agitate solution

265. The purpose of diastase in a PAS stain is to:

a. remove glycogen from cells
b. enhance the intensity of the PAS stain
c. eliminate interfering lipoprotein
d. combine with disaccharide sugars

266. One of the components demonstrated in a section stained with Luxol fast blue and counterstained with cresyl echt violet is/are:

a. melanin granules
b. glial fibers
c. Nissl substance
d. basement membranes

267. An alcian blue stain at pH 2.5 has been requested, but no alcian blue is available. Which of the following procedures could be performed to give equivalent results?

a. Luxol fast blue
b. periodic acid-Schiff
c. colloidal iron
d. mucicarmine

268. In the Weil stain, borax ferricyanide differentiates the stain by:

a. changing the pH
b. bluing the hematoxylin
c. oxidation
d. excess mordant action

269. Regressive hematoxylin staining is defined as:

a. first overstaining, then differentiating
b. staining to a desired intensity, but performing no differentiation
c. applying the hematoxylin following the counterstain
d. treating the sections with a mordant and then hematoxylin

270. Which of the following may be used to stain glycogen, polysaccharides, and glycoproteins?

a. peroxidase
b. Sudan black B
c. periodic acid-Schiff (PAS)
d. nitroblue tetrazolium (NBT)

271. A fresh solution of equal parts of potassium ferrocyanide and hydrochloric acid gives a positive reaction with:

a. iron
b. hemofuscin
c. ceroid
d. argentaffin granules

272. Bouin-fixed tissue is unsatisfactory for:

a. acid-fast stains
b. the Feulgen reaction
c. argentaffin reactions
d. mast cell demonstration

273. Which of the following procedures should be selected for the demonstration of axons?

a. Luxol fast blue
b. Bodian
c. cresyl echt violet
d. Holzer

274. A mordant in combination with a dye:

a. functions as a neutralizer
b. decolorizes on dehydration
c. acts as a differentiator
d. forms a dye lake

275. Delafield hematoxylin is most commonly aged with:

a. alcohol
b. light
c. heat
d. vacuum

276. Generally, acid dyes are differentiated in solutions that are weakly:

a. acidic
b. basic
c. neutral
d. amphoteric

277. An amphoteric substance is one that can act as a(n):

a. acid
b. base
c. salt
d. acid or base

278. The type of staining in which a weak solution of stain is used with the assumption that it will be differentially absorbed by various structures is called:

a. direct
b. indirect
c. mordant
d. adjective

279. Microscopic sections stained with H&E show a lack of nuclear staining even though the hematoxylin is well-ripened and all other solutions are fresh. Which of the following factors could explain the poor results?

a. the slides were left too long in the neutralizer
b. prolonged storage of wet tissue in unbuffered formalin
c. the pH of the hematoxylin is between 2 and 2.4
d. the embedding paraffin is too hot

280. Microscopic review of H&E-stained sections reveals that the eosin is very pale. This is most likely due to:

a. inadequate rinsing after neutralization
b. incomplete dehydration after eosin
c. the use of acetified eosin
d. improper clearing

281. The staining mechanism whereby dye adheres to the surface of structures is called:

a. absorption
b. impregnation
c. adsorption
d. orthochromasia

282. Weigert hematoxylin solution is generally unsatisfactory for use after 3 to 4:

a. hours
b. days
c. weeks
d. months

283. In a routine staining series, slides placed in xylene for clearing prior to coverslipping have an opaque appearance. This is most likely due to incomplete:

   a. neutralization
   b. dehydration
   c. deparaffinization
   d. differentiation

284. Tissue sections were stained for the recommended time with an H&E procedure using Harris hematoxylin. A quality control check shows pale nuclear staining. A likely cause of this could be:

   a. too much alum mordant in the stock hematoxylin solution
   b. excessive treatment with the bluing agent
   c. too much time in the differentiating solution
   d. prolonged dehydration and clearing

285. Dyes used for nuclear staining are:

   a. acid
   b. basic
   c. neutral
   d. amphoteric

286. A stock solution of Harris hematoxylin is being prepared for use in the routine H&E procedure. To make it an effective nuclear stain, the dye must be:

   a. amphoteric
   b. negatively charged
   c. oxidized
   d. fresh

The following items (*) have been identified as more appropriate for entry-level histotechnologists.

* 287. A fungus that can be demonstrated with various stains for acidic mucins is:

   a. *Candida albicans*
   b. *Histoplasma capsulatum*
   c. *Cryptococcus neoformans*
   d. *Coccidioides immitis*

* 288. ATPase stains are done on a muscle biopsy at pHs 9.4, 4.6, and 4.3. The slides for pH 9.4 and pH 4.3 show good differentiation of the type I and type II fibers, and although the slide done at pH 4.6 shows differentiation of the type I and type II fibers, it does not show differentiation of the type IIA and IIB fibers. This indicates that the:

   a. ammonium sulfide solution is old
   b. the pH should be modified on the 4.6 stain
   c. calcium should be omitted from the incubating solution
   d. the results of the pH 4.6 stain duplicate those of the pH 4.3 and could be omitted

* 289. A pathologic condition characterized by abnormal deposits of iron in the liver is called:

    a. hemachrosis
    b. hemochromatosis
    c. hemadostenosis
    d. hematotoxicosis

* 290. A stain is needed for a project requiring the demonstration of elastic tissue, collagen, mucin, and smooth muscle. Because tissue must be conserved, the best stain for the project is the:

    a. Verhoeff-van Gieson
    b. Masson Trichrome
    c. Mayer mucicarmine
    d. Movat pentachrome

* 291. An enzyme technique that will demonstrate denervated muscle fibers and motor end plates is the:

    a. NAD-diaphorase
    b. acid phosphatase
    c. phosphorylase
    d. alpha-naphthyl acetate esterase

* 292. Which of the following procedures will best demonstrate *Helicobacter pylori*?

    a. Fite
    b. Diff-Quik™
    c. Truant
    d. Gram

* 293. A research project requires the demonstration of lysosomes on frozen sections of muscle tissue. The best procedure would be:

    a. ATPase, pH 4.2
    b. phosphorylase
    c. acid phosphatase
    d. succinic dehydrogenase

* 294. In the PAS reaction, development of the final colored product is achieved by:

    a. oxidation of aldehyde groups
    b. extraction of diastase-sensitive structures
    c. restoration of quinoid chromophoric group
    d. cleavage of 1:2 glycol groups

* 295. Mucicarmine-positive material is noted in the cytoplasm of poorly differentiated malignant cells. This finding is indicative of a(n):

    a. adenocarcinoma
    b. squamous carcinoma
    c. leiomyosarcoma
    d. large cell lymphoma

* 296. One of the rare enzyme techniques that can be performed on paraffin sections is the:

   a. naphthol AS-D chloroacetate esterase
   b. succinic dehydrogenase
   c. alkaline phosphatase
   d. ATPase, pH 9.4

* 297. The activity of succinic dehydrogenase will be destroyed:

   a. at 37°C
   b. at pH 7.0
   c. by freezing
   d. by fixation

* 298. Acid phosphatase falls under the basic enzyme-reaction classification of:

   a. oxidoreductases
   b. transferases
   c. hydrolases
   d. isomerases

* 299. Structures that speed up the rate of enzyme reactions are known as:

   a. cofactors
   b. coenzymes
   c. substrates
   d. phosphatases

* 300. Enzymes that catalyze chemical reactions in biological systems are:

   a. metals
   b. carbohydrates
   c. proteins
   d. substrates

* 301. A procedure that demonstrates some carcinoid tumors as well as alpha cells of the pancreas is the:

   a. Fontana-Masson
   b. Warthin-Starry
   c. Grimelius
   d. periodic acid-Schiff

* 302. A patient is suspected of having McArdle disease, which is a glycogen storage disease affecting skeletal muscle. This disease is best demonstrated with which of the following techniques?

   a. alpha-naphthyl acetase esterase
   b. ATPase, pH 9.4 and 4.3
   c. acid phosphatase
   d. phosphorylase

* 303. Experiments have shown that a particular lipid fraction known as mycolic acid exists within the cell walls of:

a. *Mycobacterium tuberculosis*
b. *Pneumocystis carinii*
c. *Actinomyces bovis*
d. *Candida albicans*

* 304. Antibody molecules can belong to one of 5 immunoglobulin classes. The antibody class most frequently used in immunofluorescent and immunoenzyme staining is:

a. IgM
b. IgE
c. IgG
d. IgA

* 305. The reddish tint sometimes seen in old aluminum-hematoxylin solutions is generally caused by the:

a. evaporation of the solution
b. increased concentration of hematoxylin
c. formation of sulfuric acid from the mordant salt
d. presence of excess ammonium aluminum sulfate

* 306. In immunohistochemical procedures, excess background staining can be reduced by:

a. using whole serum antibodies
b. applying a more concentrated antibody solution
c. incubating for a shorter time in the primary antibody
d. pre-treating with nonimmune serum from the same animal species as the secondary antibody

* 307. A "hybridoma" is formed when an immunoglobulin-producing spleen cell is fused with a non-immunoglobulin–producing:

a. myeloma cell
b. liver cell
c. mesenchymal cell
d. epithelial cell

* 308. The oxidizing agent used in the Gomori chrome alum-hematoxylin-phloxine procedure for demonstrating alpha and beta cells of the pancreas is:

a. periodic acid
b. phosphotungstic acid
c. potassium permanganate
d. chromic acid

* 309. Compounds that fluoresce naturally without the use of fluorochrome dyes are said to have:

a. autofluorescence
b. secondary fluorescence
c. autoradiographic properties
d. plan apochromats

* 310. Which of the following fungi may appear as a mixture of budding yeast cells and pseudohypha elements in infected tissue?

    a. *Aspergillus*
    b. *Candida*
    c. *Histoplasma*
    d. *Cryptococcus*

* 311. Mycotic diseases that go beyond superficial or cutaneous involvement to affect vital organs and cause extensive disease and even death are referred to as:

    a. subcutaneous
    b. systemic
    c. dermatacious
    d. calcific

* 312. In a suspected case of Alzheimer's disease, a staining method that may help confirm the diagnosis is:

    a. Oil red O
    b. H&E
    c. Bielschowsky
    d. Luxol fast blue

*313. Type I muscle fibers demonstrate more positive staining results than type II fibers in oxidative histochemical procedures such as:

    a. NADH diaphorase
    b. PASH
    c. DOPA oxidase
    d. phosphorylase

* 314. An orthochromatic dye stains tissue:

    a. differently than the color of the dye itself
    b. not at all
    c. only partially
    d. the color of the color of the dye itself

* 315. The combined Gomori methods for demonstrating pancreatic alpha and beta cells involve the use of which of the following stains?

    a. Ponceau-orange G
    b. aldehyde fuchsin-phloxine B
    c. Congo red-hematoxylin
    d. chromotrope 2R-fast green

* 316. Which of the following methods should be used for the demonstration of rickettsias?

    a. Grocott
    b. Giemsa
    c. Gridley
    d. Fite

* 317. In a paraffin section, toxoplasmosis is characterized by intact cysts and/or pseudocysts containing parasites that are usually demonstrated with which procedure?

    a. hematoxylin and eosin
    b. rhodamine
    c. Fontana-Masson
    d. Ziehl-Neelsen

* 318. A malignant neoplasm characterized by gland formation and mucin production is a(n):

    a. rhabdomyosarcoma
    b. squamous carcinoma
    c. malignant melanoma
    d. adenocarcinoma

* 319. A rhabdomyosarcoma is suspected in a biopsy submitted to the laboratory. To aid in making a definitive diagnosis, a helpful stain would be the:

    a. phosphotungstic acid-hematoxylin (PTAH)
    b. Gomori aldehyde fuchsin
    c. Mayer mucicarmine
    d. Verhoeff-van Gieson

* 320. In lung tissue, coated asbestos fibers can be made more visible by staining with:

    a. Schiff reagent
    b. silver nitrate
    c. Prussian blue reaction
    d. aldehyde fuchsin

* 321. Which of the following cells is responsible for immunoglobulin production?

    a. histiocyte
    b. mast
    c. neutrophil
    d. plasma

* 322. Melanosis coli is a condition characterized by abnormal deposits of pigment that will give a positive reaction in which of the following procedures?

    a. Congo red
    b. Grimelius
    c. Schmorl
    d. von Kossa

* 323. In immunostaining, increasing the primary antibody dilution, the duration of staining, and the temperature of incubation would affect staining by:

    a. increasing both intensity and specificity
    b. decreasing both intensity and specificity
    c. increasing intensity and decreasing specificity
    d. decreasing intensity and increasing specificity

* 324. Astrocytes can be demonstrated by using the antibody that is specific for:

a. vimentin
b. S-100
c. cytokeratin
d. GFAP

* 325. Antibody diversity is due to different amino acid sequences in the variable regions of the:

a. constant region
b. light chains only
c. light and heavy chains
d. Fc fragments

* 326. Melanins are insoluble in water, alcohol, dilute acids, alkalis, and:

a. hydrogen peroxide
b. chromic acid
c. potassium permanganate
d. acetone

* 327. The specific substrate of horseradish peroxidase is:

a. diaminobenzidine
b. ethylene diamine tetraacetic acid
c. hydrogen peroxide
d. polyethylene glycol

* 328. Of the following, the best stain to demonstrate loss of muscle striations caused by dystrophic change is the:

a. Masson trichrome
b. Verhoeff-van Gieson
c. Mallory PTAH
d. Gomori trichrome

* 329. The hematoxylin-basic fuchsin-picric acid method is a technique sometimes used to demonstrate the early changes of ischemia in:

a. smooth muscle
b. cardiac muscle
c. visceral muscle
d. skeletal muscle

* 330. The amorphous transparent gel-like material that forms the bulk of extracellular content in connective tissue is known as:

a. basal lamina
b. lamina propria
c. mesenchyme
d. ground substance

* 331. Small eosinophilic inclusions found in the cytoplasm of neurons in patients infected with the rabies virus are called:

a. Barr bodies
b. Negri bodies
c. Russell bodies
d. Donovan bodies

* 332. When selecting reagents for peroxidase-anti-peroxidase (PAP) staining, the PAP complex should be prepared in the same (or a closely related) animal species as the:

a. antigen of study
b. secondary antibody
c. primary antibody
d. bridging antibody

* 333. Tumors derived from argentaffin cells are called:

a. adenomas
b. apudomas
c. carcinomas
d. sarcomas

* 334. A fungal disease characterized by pleomorphic yeast cells, narrow-based budding, and the carminophilia of the organisms is:

a. blastomycosis
b. cryptococcosis
c. histoplasmosis
d. candidiasis

* 335. A "Maltese cross" configuration is produced in tissue sections by polarization of:

a. calcium oxalate
b. uric acid
c. talcum powder
d. lipofuscin

* 336. A pigment occurring in *Plasmodium* parasites that is closely related to formalin pigment is:

a. hemoglobin
b. melanin
c. malarial
d. lipofuscin

* 337. In immunohistochemical reactions using horseradish peroxidase, a solution of hydrogen peroxide in methanol is used to:

a. block endogenous peroxidase
b. enhance background staining
c. affect reactivity of antibodies and antigens
d. intensify the coloring reaction

* 338. Luxol fast blue dye has a structural formula closely related to that of:

    a. methylene blue
    b. sky blue
    c. Nile blue sulfate
    d. alcian blue 8GX

* 339. In immunoperoxidase staining, the colored end product is formed following reduction of:

    a. a chromogenic substrate and oxidation of horseradish peroxidase
    b. hydrogen peroxide and oxidation of a chromogenic substrate
    c. a chromogenic substrate and oxidation of hydrogen peroxide
    d. hydrogen peroxide and oxidation of horseradish peroxidase

* 340. In immunohistochemical staining of formalin-fixed tissue, heat-induced epitope retrieval:

    a. increases background staining
    b. enhances primary staining
    c. is needed to demonstrate all tissue antigens
    d. has precise end-points

* 341. Which of the following non-immunological methods may be used to help identify hormone-secret-ing tumors of the pituitary gland?

    a. ammoniacal silver
    b. Luxol fast blue
    c. PAS-orange G
    d. oil red O

* 342. Following immunohistochemical staining, both the positive control and the specimen show weak staining. The most likely cause is that the:

    a. both tissues contain free antigen
    b. epitope retrieval was incorrectly done
    c. staining steps were performed in the wrong order
    d. hydrogen peroxide blocking step was omitted

* 343. A protozoan that causes neurologic disease in patients with acquired immunodeficiency syndrome (AIDS) is:

    a. *Cryptosporidium muris*
    b. *Leishmania donovani*
    c. *Giardia lamblia*
    d. *Toxoplasma gondii*

* 344. A cholecystectomy for cholelithiasis would involve the removal of a:

    a. spleen
    b. portion of liver
    c. gallbladder
    d. colon segment

* 345. Immunoperoxidase-stained tissues show reaction of red blood cells and granulocytes with the chromogenic substrate. The most likely for this explanation is that:

    a. the tissues contain antigen that reacted with the primary antiserum
    b. the specimens were improperly counterstained
    c. endogenous peroxidase was not blocked
    d. the specimens were allowed to dry during the staining procedure

* 346. "Mycoses" is the term used to describe diseases caused by:

    a. bacteria
    b. viruses
    c. fungi
    d. protozoa

* 347. Myelin contains protein, cholesterol, cerebrosides, and:

    a. fatty acids
    b. phospholipids
    c. mucoproteins
    d. endoplasmic reticulum

* 348. In the Feulgen procedure, the splitting of purines and pyrimidines from the sugar-phosphate groupings of DNA is called:

    a. autolysis
    b. synthesis
    c. hydrolysis
    d. extraction

* 349. Diseases such as malaria and leishmaniasis are caused by which of the following microorganisms?

    a. bacteria
    b. protozoa
    c. viruses
    d. fungi

* 350. Rickettsias are related to which of the following classifications of microorganisms?

    a. molds
    b. yeasts
    c. bacteria
    d. protozoa

* 351. Which of the following procedures is most suitable for demonstrating secretory granules in a carcinoid tumor?

    a. Wilder reticulin
    b. PAS-aniline blue
    c. Snook
    d. Sevier-Munger

* 352. A brown, iron-free pigment that is found in association with hemochromatosis and that stains with oil-soluble dyes in frozen sections is:

   a. hemofuscin
   b. melanin
   c. hematin
   d. bilirubin

* 353. The primary cells involved in immune responses belong to the lymphoreticular system and are found in large numbers in which of the following sites in the body?

   a. heart, lungs, liver, brain
   b. skeletal muscle, liver, pancreas, skin
   c. thymus, lymph nodes, spleen, bone marrow
   d. kidney, liver, adrenal, heart

* 354. An organism classified with bacteria, possessing both DNA and RNA, and resembling rickettsia in size and staining characteristics is:

   a. *Helicobacter pylori*
   b. *Treponema pallidum*
   c. *Leptospira interrogans*
   d. *Chlamydia* species

* 355. Fixation in a primary chromate fixative is essential if chromaffin substance is to be demonstrated by which of the following procedures?

   a. modified Steiner
   b. Gomori iron
   c. trichrome-new fuchsin
   d. Schmorl

* 356. Chromaffin-cell tumors of the adrenal gland are known as:

   a. adenomas
   b. carcinoids
   c. leiomyosarcomas
   d. pheochromocytomas

* 357. Granuloma inguinale, a venereal disease, can generally be diagnosed by using which of the following procedures?

   a. Ziehl-Neelsen
   b. Steiner
   c. Grocott
   d. Gridley

* 358. ATPase stains were performed at pH 9.4 and 4.3. Each of these stains shows large type grouping of both dark and light staining fibers. The patterns of dark and light stained fibers are reversed at the different pHs. This result is most likely due to:

   a. prolonged incubation
   b. a myopathic disease process
   c. depleted staining reagents
   d. a neuropathic disease process

* 359. A common cause of hemosiderin-laden macrophages in the lungs of elderly patients is:

   a. emphysema
   b. cardiac failure
   c. atelectasis
   d. smoking

* 360. The neuritic plaques of Alzheimer's disease can be demonstrated with the antibody that is specific for:

   a. beta-amyloid
   b. lysozyme
   c. neuron-specific enolase
   d. S-100

* 361. Which of the following will stain Paneth cells?

   a. Harris hematoxylin
   b. silver nitrate
   c. methylene blue
   d. orange G

* 362. An antibody's ability to recognize and bind with a specific protein antigen is due to its:

   a. molecular size
   b. carbohydrate structure
   c. molecular weight
   d. amino acid sequences

* 363. When evaluating fluorescent-stained cryostat sections, morphologic detail of tissues can be enhanced by examining slides using a fluorescence microscope combined with:

   a. phase contrast microscopy
   b. a polarizing microscope
   c. a dark-field microscope
   d. a tungsten light source

* 364. When staining sections for examination by fluorescence microscopy:

   a. tissue antigens are "stained" by fluorescent-labeled antiserum
   b. tissue antibodies are "stained" by fluorescent-labeled antigens
   c. fluorescent dyes are sandwiched between antigen and antibody
   d. fluorescent dyes are bound to tissue with heavy-metal mordants

* 365. In paraffin sections, hepatitis B surface antigen may be demonstrated with:

   a. Schleifstein and Parson methods
   b. Gridley and orcein methods
   c. orcein and aldehyde fuchsin methods
   d. Schleifstein and aldehyde fuchsin methods

* 366. Which of the following cells are found predominantly in gray matter of the brain and spinal cord?

    a. Schwann
    b. Reed-Sternberg
    c. ganglion
    d. astrocytes

* 367. In immunostaining, efficiency of the chromogen-substrate reaction step can be evaluated by increasing the:

    a. percentage of hydrogen peroxide in methanol
    b. time in the substrate-chromogen
    c. concentration of the chromogen
    d. number of buffer washes

* 368. The point of contact between an axon of one neuron and the dendrite of another neuron is called a(n):

    a. link
    b. synapse
    c. attachment
    d. contact

* 369. *Listeria monocytogenes*, the cause of a rare form of meningitis, can best be demonstrated in a paraffin section with which of the following staining procedures?

    a. hematoxylin and eosin
    b. Ziehl-Neelsen
    c. Grocott
    d. Gram

* 370. Beta cells of pancreatic islets and of the pituitary gland stain deep purple with which procedure?

    a. Lillie azure A-eosin B
    b. Congo red
    c. aldehyde fuchsin
    d. Gomori-Burtner

* 371. The use of heat and prolonged staining with Ziehl-Neelsen carbol fuchsin may be used to demonstrate the acid-fast characteristics of certain:

    a. proteins
    b. mucins
    c. spermatozoa
    d. lipofuscins

* 372. Immunologic staining can best be adapted for localization of surface antigens by electron microscopy following staining with:

    a. amino-ethylcarbazole
    b. colloidal gold
    c. diaminobenzidine
    d. silver nitrate

* 373. A leiomyoma is a benign tumor commonly found in the:

   a. bone
   b. uterus
   c. liver
   d. spleen

* 374. Organisms found on gastric mucosa that are the presumptive cause of gastritis, have a curved configuration, and may be stained with silver impregnation procedures are most likely:

   a. *Borrelia burgdorferi*
   b. *Treponema pallidum*
   c. *Leptospira interrogans*
   d. *Helicobacter pylori*

* 375. A method used for demonstrating acid-fast bacteria that will also demonstrate talcum powder is the:

   a. Fite
   b. Kinyoun
   c. Ziehl-Neelsen
   d. Truant

* 376. Following avidin-biotin complex (ABC) immunohistochemical staining, the cytoplasm of scattered single cells in the stroma of both positive and negative control slides appears stained. The most likely explanation is that the:

   a. cells represent avidin-containing mast cells
   b. primary antibody was applied to all slides
   c. endogenous peroxidase was not blocked
   d. staining steps were not performed in the correct order

* 377. A liver biopsy from a patient with suspected Wilson's disease shows cirrhosis. This diagnosis could be confirmed by using a rubeanic acid stain to demonstrate the presence of:

   a. bile
   b. copper
   c. lipofuscin
   d. hematoidin

* 378. The periodic acid-Schiff (PAS) procedure will stain *Coccidioides immitis* because the organisms:

   a. are argyrophilic
   b. exhibit metachromasia
   c. contain carbohydrates
   d. reduce Schiff reagent

* 379. In immunohistochemical staining, a limitation of polyclonal antibody techniques as opposed to monoclonal antibody techniques is the:

   a. greater cross-reactivity with similar antigens
   b. more difficult production of polyclonal antibodies
   c. limited availability of antisera
   d. extreme specificity of polyclonals

* 380. Which of the following pairs of adjectives describe the 2 principal defense mechanisms of the body's immune system?

    a. humoral and cell-mediated
    b. hydrolytic and cell-mediated
    c. humoral and enzymatic
    d. hydrolytic and enzymatic

* 381. The most common of the pituitary tumors are:

    a. sarcomas
    b. adenomas
    c. carcinomas
    d. teratomas

* 382. One of the most widespread and prevalent of the mycotic diseases in man is:

    a. coccidioidomycosis
    b. prototethecosis
    c. candidiasis
    d. rhinosporidiosis

* 383. One of the most useful, yet simple, techniques for identifying cell types in the pituitary gland is the:

    a. H&E
    b. Giemsa
    c. periodic acid-Schiff
    d. oil red O

* 384. In addition to being associated with a wide variety of neurons, nervous tissue is also closely associated with non-neuronal cells, including:

    a. keratinocytes and melanocytes
    b. Langerhans and Merkel cells
    c. histiocytes and mesangial cells
    d. Schwann and glial cells

* 385. Interaction between 2 single-stranded nucleic acid molecules that forms a double-stranded molecule based on the complimentary base pairing of their respective sequences is called in-situ:

    a. cloning
    b. hybridization
    c. nick translation
    d. transcription

* 386. The primary function of auxochromes in artificial dyes is to:

    a. deepen the color
    b. change the dye shade
    c. give the dye affinity for the tissue
    d. stabilize the dye compound when in solution

* 387. Two highly developed physiological properties displayed by neurons are:

    a. irritability and conductivity
    b. filtration and absorption
    c. contractility and protection
    d. surface transport and secretion

* 388. Chromaffin cells of the adrenal gland are located in the:

    a. zona glomerulosa
    b. zona reticularis
    c. zona fasciculata
    d. medulla

* 389. The refractive index of the resinous mountant used for stained sections should be approximately:

    a. 0.52 to 0.85
    b. 1.30 to 1.41
    c. 1.53 to 1.54
    d. 1.60 to 1.73

* 390. The Bielschowsky method involves double-impregnation of brain sections with silver nitrate solution. The reducing agent used in this method is:

    a. hydroquinone
    b. phenol
    c. sodium sulfite
    d. formaldehyde

* 391. All of the following microorganisms will stain with carbol-fuchsin solution EXCEPT:

    a. *Treponema pallidum*
    b. *Mycobacterium leprae*
    c. *Nocardia asteroides*
    d. Koch's bacillus

* 392. The most common basic auxochrome group encountered in dye chemistry is the:

    a. amino group ($-NH_2$)
    b. carboxyl group (–COOH)
    c. hydroxyl group (–OH)
    d. azo group (–N=N)

* 393. Nissl substance can be demonstrated by staining parallel sections before and after extraction with:

    a. diastase
    b. ribonuclease
    c. hyaluronidase
    d. deoxyribonuclease

* 394. A common acidic auxochrome is:

a. -COOH
b. -NH$_2$
c. -N=N-
d. NO$_2$

* 395. A rhabdomyosarcoma is a malignant neoplasm of:

a. smooth muscle
b. skeletal muscle
c. epithelium
d. glands

* 396. A procedure for demonstrating cytoplasmic secretory granules of the juxtaglomerular complex is:

a. Bowie
b. von Kossa
c. Mayer mucicarmine
d. Verhoeff-van Gieson

* 397. If the mucoid capsule of the fungus is intact, which of the following fungi can be differentially stained by Mayer mucicarmine?

a. *Histoplasma capsulatum*
b. *Coccidioides immitis*
c. *Cryptococcus neoformans*
d. *Candida albicans*

* 398. Although hematoxylin solutions generally require a mordant, they may be used without a mordant to demonstrate:

a. calcium
b. copper
c. lipids
d. glycogen

* 399. In reference to immunoglobulin molecules, the terms "light-" and "heavy-" chains refer to the different:

a. appearances of the chains when stained by immunofluorescence
b. molecular weight of the chains
c. amino acid sequences of the chains
d. numbers of polypeptide chains

* 400. Which of the following is a malignant neoplasm of connective tissue origin?

a. adenocarcinoma
b. glioblastoma
c. hepatocellular carcinoma
d. chondrosarcoma

* 401. "Thin" sections for electron microscopy are stained with:

   a. hematoxylin and eosin
   b. toluidine blue
   c. uranyl acetate and lead citrate
   d. fluorescein and rhodamine

* 402. The method of choice for demonstrating calcium oxalate is the:

   a. Pizzolato
   b. von Kossa
   c. Schmorl
   d. rubeanic acid

* 403. In the avidin-biotin-complex (ABC) immunohistochemical procedure:

   a. the primary antiserum is avidin-labeled
   b. no conjugation steps are involved in the reaction
   c. the ABC complex binds to biotin-labeled secondary antibody
   d. the bridging antiserum is added in excess

* 404. Ground-glass granules found in liver hepatocytes infected with the hepatitis B virus may be demonstrated with which of the following stains?

   a. Ziehl-Neelsen
   b. Brown and Brenn
   c. aldehyde fuchsin
   d. hematoxylin and eosin

* 405. Light chain monoclonality is one of the features of:

   a. B-cell non-Hodgkin's lymphoma
   b. Hodgkin's disease
   c. Castleman's disease
   d. T-cell non-Hodgkin's lymphoma

* 406. As a chromogenic substrate, aminoethylcarbazole (AEC) is preferred to diaminobenzidine (DAB) when:

   a. a permanent preparation is desired
   b. staining melanotic lesions
   c. a non-carcinogen is indicated
   d. synthetic resin mounting media are used

* 407. Which of the following procedures can be used to demonstrate *Giardia lamblia*?

   a. Giemsa
   b. Grocott
   c. Brown and Brenn
   d. Kinyoun

* 408. Malignant tumors of connective tissue are known as:

    a. carcinomas
    b. lipomas
    c. sarcomas
    d. neuromes

* 409. Which of the following procedures will demonstrate *Borrelia burgdorferi*?

    a. Fite
    b. Gridley
    c. Steiner
    d. Truant

* 410. An undifferentiated malignant neoplasm stains positive for leukocyte common antigen and negative for carcinoembryonic antigen and cytokeratin. Therefore, the origin of these malignant cells is most likely:

    a. epithelial
    b. melanocytic
    c. glandular
    d. lymphoreticular

* 411. A major reason for selecting a peroxidase-antiperoxidase (PAP) staining technique over direct or indirect conjugate methods is that, with PAP, there is(are):

    a. fewer steps involved
    b. better blockage of endogenous peroxidase
    c. increased sensitivity of antigen detection
    d. less hazard of exposure to potential carcinogens

* 412. A disorder involving excess iron deposition in tissues, with resultant tissue damage, is known as:

    a. hemosiderosis
    b. hemoglobinemia
    c. hemophilia
    d. hemochromatosis

* 413. A tumor that is thought to be associated with asbestos exposure is:

    a. dysgerminoma
    b. hepatocellular carcinoma
    c. hypernephroma
    d. mesothelioma

* 414. A cell antigen can be demonstrated by immunofluorescent staining of fresh-frozen tissues but is not visible by immunochemical staining of formalin-fixed paraffin-processed tissue. The differences in the results of the 2 methods are most likely due to:

    a. masking of antigen binding sites by fixation
    b. dilution of the primary antibody
    c. sequence of staining steps
    d. inherent procedural differences

* 415. A pathologist might choose an ATPase method to demonstrate enzyme activity in:

   a. synapses
   b. muscle fibers
   c. pancreas
   d. liver

* 416. Another name for indirect immunofluorescent staining wherein a 2-stage method is applied for identifying specific antibody-producing plasma cells within tissue is:

   a. complement incubation
   b. sandwich technique
   c. double-layer technique
   d. single-layer technique

* 417. The proteins that form the thick and thin filaments of skeletal muscle fibers are:

   a. fibrin and fibrinogen
   b. collagen and tropocollagen
   c. actin and myosin
   d. thrombin and prothrombin

* 418. A birefringent reaction product is produced following staining of calcium deposits with which of the following stains?

   a. Schmorl
   b. von Kossa
   c. dopa oxidase
   d. alizarin red S

* 419. A pigment that may be present in the portal area of the liver in association with primary biliary cirrhosis is:

   a. lipofuscin
   b. calcium
   c. hemofuscin
   d. copper

* 420. In the acid phosphatase technique, the reaction product is formed by the coupling of a diazonium salt and a(n):

   a. azo group
   b. naphthol group
   c. thymol molecule
   d. acetate salt

* 421. Neuritic plaques of Alzheimer's disease consist of abnormal cell processes, often in close proximity to deposits of:

   a. amyloid
   b. phospholipids
   c. neuromelanin
   d. astrocytes

* 422. A malignant neoplasm of connective tissue origin is classified as a(n):

   a. carcinoma
   b. sarcoma
   c. adenoma
   d. leiomyoma

* 423. Demonstrating collagen fibers with acid aniline dye-picric acid mixtures requires that the solution:

   a. be acidic
   b. be made fresh
   c. contain oxalic acid
   d. use ethanol as the solvent

* 424. A monoclonal antibody that has good specificity for demonstrating amelanotic melanomas is:

   a. HMB-45
   b. S-100
   c. Factor VIII
   d. calcitonin

* 425. The area of the brain that usually contains neuromelanin is the:

   a. pons
   b. substantia nigra
   c. medulla
   d. hypothalamus

* 426. Oxytocin and antidiuretic hormone are 2 of the hormones secreted by the:

   a. pancreas
   b. thyroid
   c. pineal body
   d. pituitary

* 427. The diagnosis of Alzheimer's disease is based on the presence of neurofibrillary tangles and neuritic plaques in the:

   a. spinal cord
   b. cortex
   c. medulla oblongata
   d. cerebellum

* 428. Silver nitrate is not available to perform a requested basement membrane stain. Another method that can be used is:

   a. alcian blue-aldehyde fuchsin
   b. Masson trichrome
   c. periodic acid-Schiff
   d. Weigert resorcin fuchsin

* 429. A trainee about to perform a Feulgen reaction reports that no Feulgen reagent can be found in the lab. The trainee should be told to look instead for which of the following reagents?

a. Schmorl
b. van Gieson
c. Schiff
d. Fouchet

* 430. The HMB-45 antibody is associated with the demonstration of:

a. melanin
b. hemoglobin
c. hemosiderin
d. lipofuscin

* 431. Microscopic evaluation of a section of brain stained with the Holzer technique should show:

a. dark blue myelin
b. blue to purple glial fibers
c. black axons and dendrites
d. violet Nissl substance

* 432. Microscopic evaluation of an auramine-rhodamine–stained control section shows minute, shiny, orange structures against a dark background. This control can be considered positive for:

a. *Legionella*
b. *Treponema*
c. *Candida*
d. *Mycobacterium*

* 433. A histochemical procedure for demonstrating non-specific esterase will show the enzyme's:

a. structure
b. origin
c. activity
d. protein

* 434. An H&E-stained section is microscopically evaluated for quality. Which of the following is sufficient criterion for rejection of the slides?

a. crisp blue nuclei
b. pale pink to gray collagen
c. well-defined chromatin
d. bright pink-red erythrocytes

* 435. The terms acidophilic, basophilic, and sudanophilic reflect the ability of various cellular components to bind with:

a. eosin, phloxine, and Sudan IV
b. eosin, hematoxylin, and Sudan black B
c. hematoxylin, carmine, and oil red O
d. methyl green, hematoxylin, and Sudan III

* 436. In the coupling method for alkaline phosphatase, the naphthol must be coupled with which of the following?

    a. acetate
    b. formazan
    c. diazonium
    d. phenylalanine

* 437. PTAH stains would be LEAST useful in differentiating:

    a. fibrin
    b. rhabdomyosarcomas
    c. gliosis
    d. pheochromocytomas

* 438. *Pneumocystis carinii* is best demonstrated by:

    a. hematoxylin and eosin
    b. periodic acid-Schiff
    c. methenamine-silver
    d. Dieterle technique

* 439. A control section used in a Grocott methenamine-silver procedure is known to contain *Aspergillus* species. Microscopic evaluation reveals dense, black walls of the hyphae, with pale gray internal structures and a green background. This result should be considered:

    a. excellent
    b. minimally acceptable
    c. poor because the organisms are understained
    d. unacceptable because the wrong technique was used

* 440. Consider the following staining results:

    - PAS is negative
    - Alcian blue pH 2.5 is positive
    - Colloidal iron is positive

The stained sections most likely contain:

    a. neutral mucopolysaccharides
    b. basement membrane material
    c. fungal organisms
    d. acid mucopolysaccharides

* 441. Just before use in the routine H&E procedure, acetic acid may be added to stock Harris hematoxylin to:

   a. improve selectivity of the stain for chromatin
   b. facilitate subsequent cytoplasmic staining
   c. increase dye lake formation
   d. avoid long bluing times

* 442. Schmorl technique depends upon:

   a. ferric iron reduction
   b. colloidal iron absorption
   c. the argyrophil substance present
   d. bilirubin oxidation

* 443. Control material to be used with Best carmine technique can be found in the:

   a. kidney
   b. liver
   c. testes
   d. colon

* 444. A section stained with Fouchet reagent shows discrete emerald-green globules. This indicates the presence of:

   a. melanosomes
   b. hemosiderin
   c. bilirubin
   d. acid hematin

* 445. The differential diagnosis of a lymph node biopsy includes metastatic melanoma. The tissue should be:

   a. available for acid phosphatase
   b. frozen for an enzyme profile
   c. fixed for demonstration of HMB-45 antigen
   d. prepared for cytologic examination and fixed in Bouin fluid

* 446. A student submits a control section of appendix on which a Schmorl stain has been done. No positive granules can be identified microscopically. Analysis of the procedure reveals the following:
   1 - ferric chloride and potassium ferrocyanide
      were used in the freshly prepared staining solution
   2 - the sections were stained for 10 minutes in the solution

   The problem can be identified as the fact that:

   a. appendix is not a good control for argentaffin cells
   b. the staining solution should have contained potassium ferricyanide
   c. the staining solution should have been aged
   d. Schmorl technique does not demonstrate granules

* 447. The microscopic quality control check of an H&E-stained section reveals lightly stained nuclei lacking sharp chromatin detail. These results are an indication of:

a. poor fixation
b. poor processing
c. outdated bluing reagent
d. contaminated mountant

* 448. DNA is NOT demonstrated on microscopic sections of a lymph node treated for 1 hour with 1 N hydrochloric acid at 60°C, followed by staining with Schiff reagent for 1 hour. The most likely explanation for this is:

a. the omission of a periodate oxidation step
b. excessive hydrolysis of the nuclei
c. the use of hydrochloric acid for pretreatment
d. excessive staining time in Schiff reagent

* 449. In an immunoperoxidase procedure, the primary antibody used is a mouse monoclonal anti-Leu-4. Which secondary antibody would be appropriate?

a. goat anti-rabbit
b. goat anti-mouse
c. bovine serum albumin
d. biotinylated anti-rabbit

* 450. In a Verhoeff-van Gieson stain, the adventitia of large arteries stain similarly to:

a. elastin
b. epithelium
c. nuclei
d. collagen

* 451. The staining of fat by Sudan black B is due to the:

a. chemical linkage of fat and dye
b. adsorption of dye by fat
c. solubility of dye in fat
d. precipitation of dye in fat

* 452. Refer to the following diagram:

$$NH_3^+ - \underset{\underset{H}{|}}{\overset{\overset{R}{|}}{C}} - COOH$$

The amphoteric amino acid shown in the above diagram:

a. migrates in an electrical field to the positive pole
b. is appropriately charged for eosin staining
c. is at the isoelectric point
d. is receptive to basic dyes

* 453. One difference between rotary and linear automatic stainers is that rotary stainers:

    a. require a different solution in each container
    b. require the use of regressive dyes
    c. permit different times in each compartment
    d. permit staining of thicker sections

* 454 Which of the following procedures is most specific for the identification of melanomas in paraffin sections?
    a. DOPA reaction
    b. Fontana-Masson
    c. Warthin-Starry, pH 3.1
    d. immunohistochemistry for HMB-45

* 455. If you purchase an unlabeled monoclonal antibody to a specific antigen, the second antibody applied most commonly is:

    a. rabbit anti-mouse
    b. rabbit anti-goat
    c. goat anti-human
    d. mouse anti-human

* 456. Pyroninophilia indicates the presence of:

    a. deoxyribonucleic acid
    b. ribonucleic acid
    c. ribonuclease
    d. mitochondria

* 457. The auxochrome is the group present in dyes that:

    a. acts as an oxidizer
    b. is associated with color
    c. is responsible for forming ionic bonds
    d. features double bonds involving carbon and/or nitrogen

* 458. Simultaneous coupling is a technique used in:

    a. acid mucopolysaccharide demonstration
    b. immunofluorescence
    c. enzyme histochemistry
    d. electron microscopy

* 459. The Color Index printed on the label of a stain bottle refers to the:

    a. purity of the stain
    b. percentage of the stain present
    c. maximum absorption peak
    d. standard identification number

* 460. A staining reaction that depends upon ionization of both the dye and the material on which the dye is precipitated is termed:

 a. mordant staining
 b. indirect staining
 c. absorption
 d. adsorption

* 461. The naphthol AS-D chloroacetate esterase technique is useful in identifying which of the following cells?

 a. fibroblasts
 b. monocytes
 c. neutrophils
 d. lymphocytes

* 462. Microscopic examination of a Carnoy-fixed control section of kidney known to contain amyloid fails to show green birefringence following Congo red staining. This finding is:

 a. correct for Congo red stains
 b. indicative of a staining problem
 c. the result of improper fixation
 d. typical of freshly cut control sections

* 463. Pure methyl green used at a slightly acid pH is considered a specific stain for:

 a. aldehydes
 b. polysaccharides
 c. DNA
 d. RNA

* 464. The Weil stain will demonstrate which structure of the eye?

 a. cornea
 b. iris
 c. optic nerve
 d. sclera

* 465. Specific stains for prostate cancer are prostate-specific antigen and:

 a. non-specific esterase
 b. acid phosphatase
 c. ATPase
 d. dehydrogenase

* 466. The type of staining in which tissue soaks up dye and is completely penetrated by it is called:

 a. adsorption
 b. absorption
 c. vital
 d. routine

* 467. The most useful method by which dyes can be checked for impurities and the presence of other dyes is known as:

a. chromatography
b. titration
c. nitrogen assay
d. optical identification

* 468. Microscopic examination shows no pink staining on an H&E-stained section. To isolate the problem, the first step is to:

a. repeat the dehydration step
b. recut and restain the sections
c. check the type of eosin
d. check the pH of the eosin

Staining Answer Key

The following items have been identified as appropriate for both entry level histologic technicians and histotechnologists.

1. c	36. b	71. d	106. d
2. c	37. c	72. c	107. d
3. c	38. b	73. b	108. c
4. a	39. a	74. c	109. c
5. b	40. b	75. c	110. c
6. d	41. b	76. c	111. d
7. b	42. c	77. d	112. d
8. d	43. d	78. b	113. b
9. d	44. c	79. d	114. c
10. c	45. c	80. b	115. a
11. d	46. b	81. c	116. d
12. c	47. c	82. b	117. a
13. a	48. b	83. d	118. b
14. b	49. c	84. c	119. c
15. b	50. b	85. c	120. a
16. c	51. a	86. a	121. c
17. b	52. b	87. b	122. d
18. b	53. c	88. b	123. c
19. c	54. c	89. c	124. d
20. a	55. c	90. c	125. c
21. d	56. d	91. c	126. b
22. c	57. d	92. b	127. c
23. b	58. c	93. b	128. a
24. d	59. d	94. c	129. c
25. c	60. b	95. a	130. b
26. a	61. a	96. a	131. c
27. c	62. d	97. a	132. d
28. b	63. a	98. c	133. b
29. d	64. c	99. b	134. d
30. a	65. b	100. a	135. a
31. b	66. c	101. c	136. c
32. a	67. c	102. d	137. b
33. b	68. b	103. a	138. b
34. d	69. d	104. c	139. b
35. b	70. c	105. c	140. a

141. a	178. d	215. c	252. d
142. b	179. b	216. b	253. c
143. c	180. a	217. b	254. d
144. a	181. a	218. b	255. d
145. a	182. a	219. a	256. d
146. c	183. b	220. b	257. a
147. c	184. c	221. c	258. c
148. b	185. a	222. c	259. c
149. c	186. a	223. a	260. b
150. c	187. a	224. c	261. d
151. d	188. a	225. d	262. d
152. b	189. d	226. b	263. d
153. a	190. d	227. b	264. d
154. b	191. d	228. b	265. d
155. c	192. a	229. d	266. c
156. b	193. b	230. d	267. c
157. a	194. d	231. c	268. c
158. b	195. c	232. b	269. a
159. b	196. a	233. a	270. c
160. c	197. d	234. c	271. a
161. c	198. c	235. a	272. b
162. a	199. c	236. b	273. b
163. a	200. c	237. d	274. d
164. d	201. b	238. d	275. b
165. d	202. c	239. a	276. b
166. c	203. d	240. a	277. d
167. d	204. c	241. d	278. a
168. d	205. a	242. b	279. b
169. c	206. b	243. a	280. a
170. c	207. c	244. a	281. c
171. a	208. d	245. b	282. b
172. c	209. b	246. c	283. b
173. d	210. d	247. c	284. c
174. c	211. d	248. a	285. b
175. d	212. b	249. c	286. c
176. b	213. a	250. d	
177. b	214. a	251. d	

The following items (*) have been identified as more appropriate for the entry level histotechnologists.

* 287. c	* 322. c	* 357. b	* 392. a
* 288. b	* 323. a	* 358. d	* 393. b
* 289. b	* 324. d	* 359. b	* 394. a
* 290. d	* 325. c	* 360. a	* 395. b
* 291. d	* 326. d	* 361. d	* 396. a
* 292. b	* 327. c	* 362. d	* 397. c
* 293. c	* 328. c	* 363. a	* 398. b
* 294. c	* 329. b	* 364. a	* 399. b
* 295. a	* 330. d	* 365. c	* 400. d
* 296. a	* 331. b	* 366. d	* 401. c
* 297. d	* 332. c	* 367. b	* 402. b
* 298. c	* 333. b	* 368. b	* 403. c
* 299. a	* 334. b	* 369. d	* 404. c
* 300. c	* 335. c	* 370. c	* 405. a
* 301. c	* 336. c	* 371. d	* 406. b
*302. d	* 337. a	* 372. b	* 407. a
* 303. a	* 338. d	* 373. b	* 408. c
* 304. c	* 339. b	* 374. d	* 409. c
* 305. c	* 340. b	* 375. d	* 410. d
* 306. d	* 341. c	* 376. a	* 411. c
* 307. a	* 342. b	* 377. b	* 412. d
* 308. c	* 343. d	* 378. c	* 413. d
* 309. a	* 344. c	* 379. a	* 414. a
* 310. d	* 345. c	* 380. a	* 415. b
* 311. b	* 346. c	* 381. b	* 416. c
* 312. c	* 347. b	* 382. c	* 417. c
* 313. a	* 348. c	* 383. c	* 418. d
* 314. d	* 349. b	* 384. d	* 419. d
* 315. b	* 350. d	* 385. b	* 420. b
* 316. b	* 351. d	* 386. c	* 421. a
* 317. a	* 352. a	* 387. a	* 422. b
* 318. d	* 353. c	* 388. d	* 423. a
* 319. a	* 354. d	* 389. c	* 424. a
* 320. c	* 355. d	* 390. d	* 425. b
* 321. d	* 356. d	* 391. a	* 426. d

* 427. b   * 438. c   * 449. b   *460. d
* 428. c   * 439. a   * 450. d   *461. c
* 429. c   * 440. d   * 451. c   *462. b
* 430. a   * 441. a   * 452. b   *463. c
* 431. b   * 442. a   * 453. c   *464. c
* 432. d   * 443. b   * 454. d   *465. b
* 433. c   * 444. c   * 455. a   *466. b
* 434. b   * 445. c   * 456. b   *467. a
* 435. b   * 446. b   * 457. c   *468. d
* 436. c   * 447. a   *458. c
* 437. d   * 448. b   *459. d

Chapter 14

Image-Based Questions

The following items have been identified as appropriate for both entry-level histologic technicians and histotechnologists.

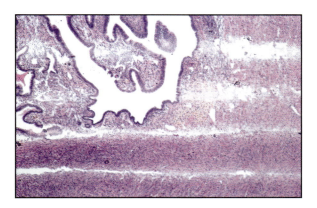

Image 14.1

1. Corrective action for the artifact in Image 14.1 should include:

   a. reducing waterbath temperature
   b. prolonging fixation in formalin
   c. tightening microtome clamps
   d. reorienting the tissue in the block

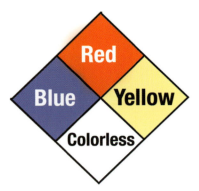

2. The number 4 placed in the red quadrant of the
National Fire Protection Association (NFPA) diamond in Image 14.2 would indicate a chemical
that:

   a. can cause death on short exposure
   b. is very reactive and may detonate
   c. can be easily ignited at room temperature
   d. is a very strong oxidizer

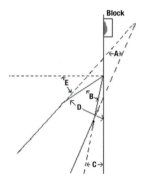

Image 14.3
This image pertains to questions 3 and 4.

3. If angle C in Image 14.3 is increased, the result may be:

   a. alternate thick and thin sections
   b. chatter or undulations in the sections
   c. vertical lines in the sections
   d. lifting of sections from the knife

4. When alternating thick and thin sections are obtained, which of the following would most likely
correct the problem?

   a. increase angle B
   b. increase angle C
   c. decrease angle D
   d. increase angle E

Image 14.4

STATION	SOLUTION	MINUTES	TEMPERATURE
1	10% NBF	45	26°C
2	10% NBF	45	26°C
3	70% Ethanol	45	26°C
4	80% Ethanol	45	26°C
5	95% Ethanol	45	26°C
6	95% Ethanol	45	26°C
7	100% Ethanol	45	26°C
8	100% Ethanol	45	26°C
9	100% Ethanol	45	26°C
10	Xylene	45	26°C
11	Xylene	45	26°C
12	Paraffin	45	62°C
13	Paraffin	45	62°C
14	Paraffin	45	62°C

5. Multiple sections of spleen have been processed in a closed system tissue processor using the program shown in Image 14.4. The tissue is brittle. In order to avoid this problem in the future, the following program changes should be made:

    a. increase the time in 10% NBF
    b. change station 3 to 60% ethanol
    c. change station 9 to xylene
    d. reduce the temperature in stations 1 through 11

Image 14.5

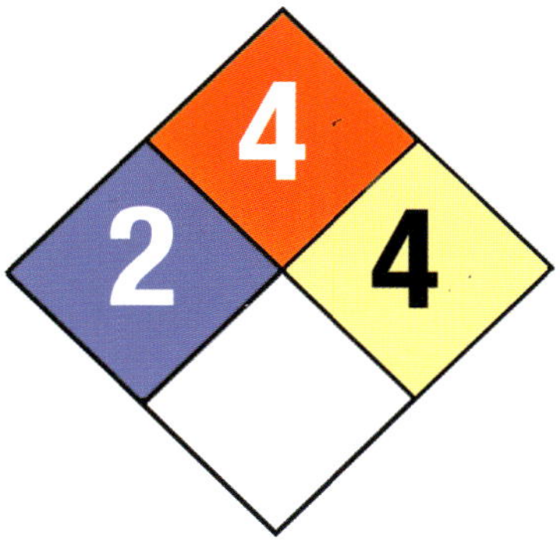

6. The symbol in Image 14.5 would apply to which of the following fixatives/components?

    a. B5
    b. formalin
    c. picric acid
    d. Carnoy

7. The symbol (Image 14.6) posted in an area would indicate which of the following hazards?

   a. electrical
   b. radiation
   c. biohazard
   d. explosive

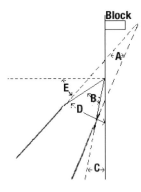

Image 14.7

This image pertains to questions 8 and 9.

8. Using Image 14.7, identify the angles shown.

   a. A is the wedge angle; B is the bevel angle; C is the clearance angle.
   b. B is the wedge angle; C is the bevel angle; A is the clearance angle.
   c. C is the wedge angle; A is the bevel angle; B is the clearance angle.
   d. B is the wedge angle; A is the bevel angle; C is the clearance angle.

9. Referring to Image 14.7, identify angle B:

   a. rake angle
   b. bevel angle
   c. wedge angle
   d. cutting angle

10. When this symbol (Image 14.8) is posted, material stored in the area requires:

    a. shielding or containment techniques
    b. that employees wear personal protective equipment around it
    c. storage in a biological safety cabinet
    d. protection from an ignition source

Image 14.9

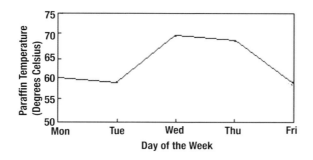

11. According to the graph of paraffin bath temperatures shown in Image 14.9, how many days of the week may reveal problems in microtomy? The melting point of the paraffin is 56° to 58°C.

    a. none
    b. one
    c. two
    d. three

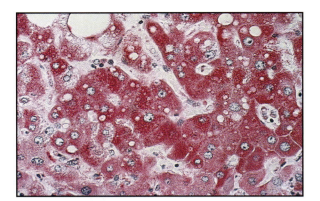

Image 14.10

This image pertains to questions 12–18.

12. The tissue shown in Image 14.10 is:

    a. spleen
    b. lung
    c. brain
    d. liver

13. The technique shown in Image 14.10 is the:

    a. oil red O
    b. Masson trichrome
    c. Congo red
    d. periodic acid-Schiff

14. The oxidizer used in the technique illustrated in Image 14.10 is:

    a. chromic acid
    b. periodic acid
    c. potassium permanganate
    d. sodium metabisulfite

15. The technique illustrated in Image 14.10 depends upon the:

    a. formation of aldehydes
    b. presence of the carboxylate group
    c. presence of the sulfate group
    d. digestion of hyaluronidase

16. False-positive results may occur with the technique illustrated in Image 14.10 if the tissue
    is fixed in:

    a. glutaraldehyde
    b. buffered formaldehyde
    c. Bouin solution
    d. absolute alcohol

17. The technique illustrated in Image 14.10 is used for the demonstration of:

    a. Nissl substance
    b. *Mycobacterium tuberculosis*
    c. glycogen
    d. reducing substances

18. The technique illustrated in Image 14.10 demonstrates:

    a. sulfated acid mucopolysaccharides
    b. carboxylated acid mucopolysaccharides
    c. neutral polysaccharides
    d. chondroitin sulfate

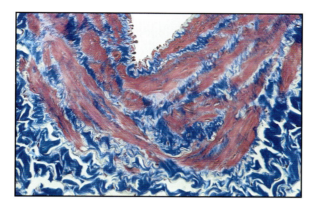

Image 14.11
This image pertains to questions 19–23.

19. The preferred fixative for the technique shown in Image 14.11 is:

    a. neutral buffered formalin
    b. Bouin solution
    c. absolute alcohol
    d. B-5 solution

20. The material stained blue in Image 14.11 is:

    a. collagen
    b. muscle
    c. cartilage
    d. reticulin

21. Before performing the technique illustrated in Image 14.11, formalin-fixed tissue must be mordanted in which of the following solutions?

    a. Zenker
    b. Carnoy
    c. Bouin
    d. B-5

22. The material stained red in Image 14.11 is:

   a. collagen
   b. smooth muscle
   c. cartilage
   d. striated muscle

23. The technique shown in Image 14.11 is often used in the diagnosis of:

   a. pancreatic islet cell diseases
   b. mycotic diseases
   c. blood vessel invasion by tumor
   d. cirrhosis of the liver

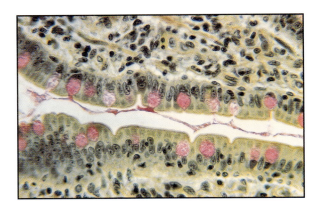

Image 14.12
This image pertains to questions 24–28.

24. Stained red-pink in Image 14.12 are:

   a. Kulchitsky cells
   b. Paneth granules
   c. lipid droplets
   d. goblet cells

25. The technique shown in Image 14.12 is the:

   a. Mayer mucicarmine
   b. oil red O
   c. Congo red
   d. Alizarin red S

26. The technique shown in Image 14.12 is used for the demonstration of:

   a. epithelial mucins
   b. connective tissue mucins
   c. glycogen
   d. neutral polysaccharides

27. The stain demonstrated in Image 14.12 can also be used to demonstrate:

   a. *Coccidioides immitis*
   b. *Candida albicans*
   c. *Cryptococcus neoformans*
   d. *Histoplasma capsulatum*

28. The number of red stained cells in Image 14.12 indicates that the tissue is most likely from the:

    a. esophagus
    b. stomach
    c. small intestine
    d. colon

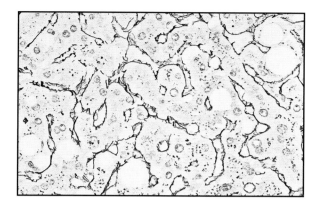

Image 14.13

This image pertains to questions 29–34.

29. The technique shown in Image 14.13 demonstrates:

    a. basement membranes
    b. elastic fibers
    c. reducing substances
    d. reticulin

30. The first step in the technique illustrated in Image 14.13 is:

    a. sensitization
    b. oxidation
    c. reduction
    d. digestion

31. In the technique illustrated in Image 14.13, formaldehyde is used as a(n):

    a. sensitizer
    b. oxidizer
    c. reducer
    d. toner

32. The preferred control tissue for the technique illustrated in Image 14.13 is:

    a. pancreas
    b. kidney
    c. uterus
    d. liver

33. In the technique illustrated in Image 14.13, a metallic solution such as uranyl nitrate or ferric ammonium sulfate is used for:

    a. oxidation
    b. sensitization
    c. reduction
    d. toning

34. The pattern of staining seen in Image 14.13 is common in tissue from which of the following organs?

    a. pancreas
    b. liver
    c. kidney
    d. lymph node

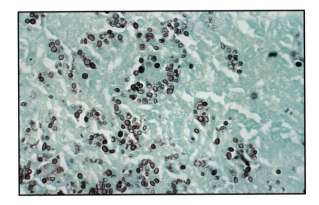

Image 14.14
This image pertains to questions 35–40.

35. The black-stained structures demonstrated in Image 14.14 are most likely:

    a. calcium granules
    b. carbon pigment
    c. fungi
    d. urate crystals

36. The technique demonstrated in Image 14.14 is the:

    a. Gram
    b. Grocott
    c. Giemsa
    d. Grimelius

37. Chromic acid is traditionally used in the technique illustrated in Image 14.14 to:

    a. oxidize polysaccharides to aldehydes
    b. prevent overoxidation of weak polysaccharides
    c. mordant formaldehyde-fixed tissue
    d. begin impregnation

38. Overstaining for the black structures shown in Image 14.14 would be indicated by:

    a. nonspecific silver precipitation
    b. crisp black cell walls
    c. the lack of visible internal structure
    d. the lack of visible hyphae

39. The black-stained structures shown in Image 14.14 are most likely:

    a. calcium spherules
    b. *Coccidioides immitis*
    c. *Histoplasma capsulatum*
    d. urate crystals

40. The term used to designate disease produced by the organisms shown in Image 14.14 is:

    a. inflammation
    b. mycosis
    c. viral
    d. parasitic

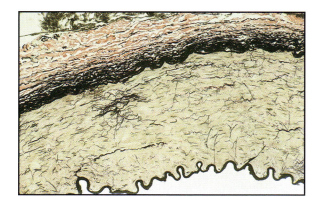

Image 14.15
This image pertains to questions 41–46.

41. The counterstain for the procedure shown in Image 14.15 contains:

    a. metanil yellow
    b. basic fuchsin
    c. picric acid
    d. orange G

42. The technique shown in Image 14.15 is the:

    a. aldehyde fuchsin
    b. Wilder silver nitrate
    c. Verhoeff–van Gieson
    d. von Kossa

43. The fibers in Image 14.15 are stained black by:

    a. iron hematoxylin
    b. aluminum hematoxylin
    c. methenamine silver
    d. diamine silver

44. The black-stained fibers in Image 14.15 are:

    a. reticulin
    b. axons
    c. basement membranes
    d. elastic

45. The red-stained material in Image 14.15 is:

    a. smooth muscle
    b. collagen
    c. cartilage
    d. striated muscle

46. The tissue shown in Image 14.15 is a(n):

    a. capillary
    b. vein
    c. elastic artery
    d. muscular artery

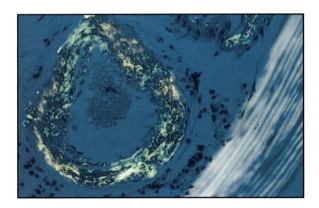

Image 14.16
This image pertains to questions 47–53.

47. The technique shown in Image 14.16 is known as:

    a. dark-field
    b. polarization
    c. phase contrast
    d. dichroism

48. The material on the right that is silvery-white in Image 14.16 is:

   a. calcium
   b. amyloid
   c. muscle
   d. collagen

49. The staining technique most likely used in Image 14.16 is the:

   a. PAS
   b. Congo red
   c. crystal violet
   d. mucicarmine

50. Another method that can be used to demonstrate the component stained green in Image 14.16 is:

   a. auramine-rhodamine
   b. aldehyde fuchsin
   c. thioflavin T
   d. mucicarmine

51. What micrometer thickness is preferred for the technique shown in Image 14.16?

   a. 2 to 3
   b. 4 to 6
   c. 8 to 10
   d. 12 to 15

52. Prolonged storage of cut control sections for the technique shown in Image 14.16 will:

   a. cause loss of positivity
   b. improve polarization
   c. result in increased background
   d. enhance staining of old deposits

53. The green component in Image 14.16 is most likely:

   a. amyloid
   b. glycogen
   c. collagen
   d. calcium

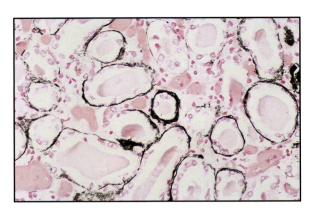

Image 14.17

This image pertains to questions 54–57.

54. The substance stained black in Image 14.17 is most likely:

   a. iron
   b. calcium
   c. hematin
   d. bile

55. The technique shown in Image 14.17 is most likely the:

   a. Schmorl
   b. Gomori-Burtner
   c. Steiner
   d. von Kossa

56. Another technique that could be used to demonstrate the pigment stained black in Image 14.17 is the:

   a. Schmorl
   b. Fontana-Masson
   c. alizarin red S
   d. rhodanine

57. The method shown in Image 14.17 uses silver to demonstrate:

   a. calcium
   b. phosphates
   c. aldehydes
   d. urates

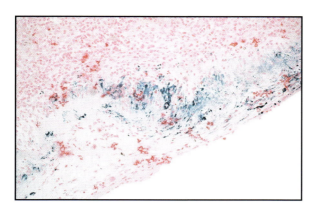

Image 14.18

This image pertains to questions 58–61.

58. The red material seen in Image 14.18 is most likely:

   a. lipid
   b. stain precipitate
   c. hemofuscin
   d. mycobacteria

59. The blue-stained substance in Image 14.18 is demonstrated with a method using hydrochloric acid and:

   a. colloidal iron
   b. potassium ferricyanide
   c. potassium ferrocyanide
   d. methylene blue

60. The end-product of the reaction demonstrated in Image 14.18 is:

   a. ferric ferrocyanide
   b. ferrous ferricyanide
   c. potassium ferrocyanide
   d. potassium ferricyanide

61. The technique demonstrated in Image 14.18 is used to demonstrate:

   a. reducing substances
   b. hemosiderin
   c. hemoglobin
   d. ferrous ions

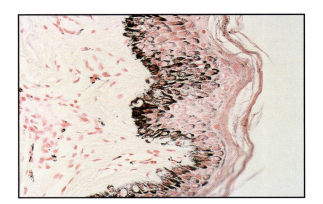

Image 14.19

This image pertains to questions 62–67.

62. The tissue in Image 14.19 is:

    a. spleen
    b. esophagus
    c. cervix
    d. skin

63. The technique shown in Image 14.19 is most likely the:

    a. Grocott
    b. von Kossa
    c. Fontana-Masson
    d. Gomori-Burtner

64. The substance stained black in Image 14.19 is most likely:

    a. calcium
    b. melanin
    c. urate crystals
    d. anthracotic pigment

65. The technique shown in Image 14.19 demonstrates substances that are:

    a. argyrophilic
    b. reducing
    c. oxidizing
    d. metachromatic

66. Another technique that can be used to demonstrate the material stained black in Image 14.19 is:

    a. Sevier-Munger
    b. von Kossa
    c. Schmorl
    d. PAS

67. The cells containing the black-stained material in Image 14.19 are found in the:

    a. epidermis
    b. dermis
    c. hypodermis
    d. keratin

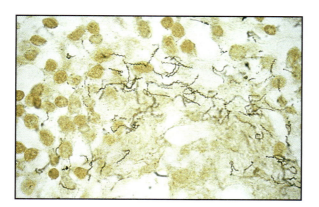

Image 14.20
This image pertains to questions 68–72.

68. The black-stained structures in Image 14.20 are most likely:

    a. mycobacteria
    b. staphlococci
    c. rickettsia
    d. spirochetes

69. The black-stained structures in Image 14.20 most likely were stained with which of the following procedures:

    a. Truant
    b. Steiner
    c. Grocott
    d. Gram

70. Poor results might be obtained with the procedure illustrated in Image 14.20 if the:

    a. tissue was fixed in neutral buffered formalin
    b. reducing solution contained hydroquinone
    c. glassware used was not chemically cleaned
    d. sections are heated at any step

71. The structures in Image 14.20 stain black with silver because of the:

    a. subsequent application of a chemical reducing agent
    b. inherent ability of the organism to reduce silver
    c. specificity of the method for the organism
    d. formation of ionic bonds

72. The organism stained black in Image 14.20 is most likely:

    a. *Helicobacter pylori*
    b. *Treponema pallidum*
    c. *Mycobacterium leprae*
    d. *Pseudomonas aeruginosa*

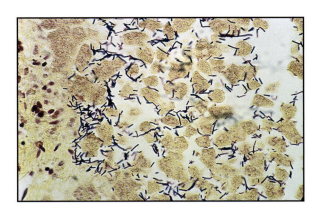

73. The blue-black structures shown in Image 14.21 are most likely:

    a. mycobacteria
    b. spirochetes
    c. bacilli
    d. hyphae

74. The staining procedure illustrated in Image 14.21 is most likely the:

    a. Grimelius
    b. Gridley
    c. Giemsa
    d. Gram

75. The structures stained blue-black in Image 14.21 are:

    a. gram-positive
    b. gram-negative
    c. acid-fast
    d. argentaffin

76. The blue-black structures in Image 14.21 are stained by:

    a. Gallego solution
    b. methylene blue
    c. crystal violet
    d. basic fuchsin

77. The rose-stained structures in Image 14.22 are most likely:

    a. calcium
    b. amyloid
    c. fungi
    d. amoeba

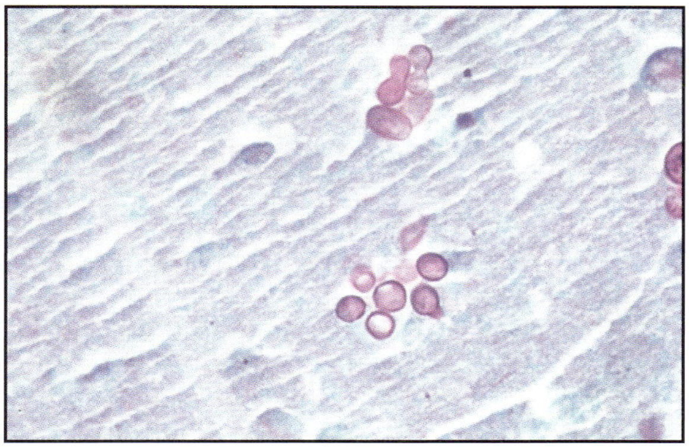

Image 14.22
This image pertains to questions 77–84.

78. The procedure illustrated in Image 14.22 is most likely the:

    a. PAS
    b. Feulgen
    c. Gridley
    d. Congo Red

79. The procedure illustrated in Image 14.22 depends upon the formation of:

    a. ketones
    b. aldehydes
    c. amino groups
    d. hydrogen bonds

80. The structures stained rose in Image 14.22 are also demonstrated frequently by which of the following stains?

    a. Congo Red
    b. Giemsa
    c. Gram
    d. Grocott

81. The technique demonstrated in Image 14.22 depends upon oxidation with:

    a. phosphomolybdic acid
    b. potassium permanganate
    c. periodic acid
    d. sodium iodate

82. The illustration in Image 14.22 shows the results of:

    a. an improper knife angle
    b. the wrong choice of fixative
    c. flotation on a cold water bath
    d. incorrect facing of the block

83. The primary staining reagent in the procedure illustrated in Image 14.22 is a reduced solution of:

    a. acid fuchsin
    b. basic fuchsin
    c. crystal violet
    d. thionin

84. The viability of the primary staining solution used in the procedure illustrated in Image 14.22 can be checked with:

   a. acetic acid
   b. a pH meter
   c. formaldehyde
   d. sodium bisulfite

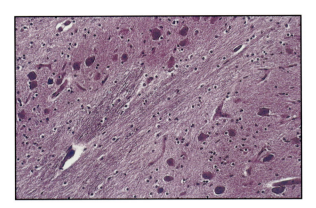

Image 14.23
This image pertains to questions 85–87.

85. The stain illustrated in Image 14.23 is a poor Luxol fast blue-cresyl echt violet stain. For this stain, cresyl echt violet should stain ONLY the:

   a. glial cells
   b. myelin sheath
   c. nuclei and Nissl substance
   d. neurofibrillary tangles

86. The results in the illustration in Image 14.23 of a Luxol fast blue-cresyl echt violet stain are poor. The primary problem is most likely the result of:

   a. improperly prepared Luxol fast blue
   b. incorrect temperature for staining
   c. underdifferentiation of the Luxol fast blue
   d. nonacidification of the cresyl echt violet

87. The primary problem shown in the illustration in Image 14.23 of a Luxol fast blue-cresyl echt violet stain could most likely be corrected by:

   a. verifying the addition of acetic acid to the cresyl echt violet
   b. decreasing the temperature of the cresyl echt violet staining
   c. checking the preparation of the Luxol fast blue solution
   d. increasing the time of differentiation of the Luxol fast blue

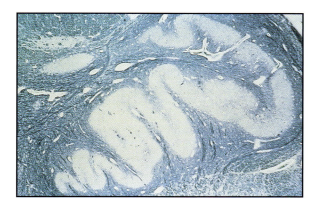

Image 14.24
This image pertains to questions 88–93.

88. The technique shown in Image 14.24 is the:

    a. Bodian
    b. Luxol fast blue
    c. Prussian blue
    d. Bielschowski

89. The material stained blue in Image 14.24 is:

    a. amyloid
    b. iron
    c. myelin
    d. Nissl substance

90. The specific section of central nervous system tissue shown in Image 14.24 is the:

    a. cerebellum
    b. medulla
    c. pons
    d. cerebral cortex

91. Another technique that could be used to demonstrate the substance stained blue in Image 14.24 is that of:

    a. Holmes
    b. Bodian
    c. Holzer
    d. Weil

92. The staining technique demonstrated in Image 14.24 used a(n):

    a. polychrome dye
    b. iron hematoxylin lake
    c. silver proteinate solution
    d. sulfonated copper phthalocyanine dye

93. The white structure seen in Image 14.24 is the:

    a. olivary nucleus
    b. choroid plexus
    c. Purkinje cell layer
    d. corticospinal tract

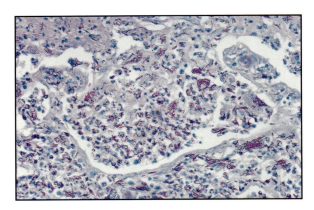

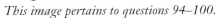

Image 14.25

This image pertains to questions 94–100.

94. The staining technique illustrated in Image 14.25 is most likely that of:

   a. Gram
   b. Giemsa
   c. Kinyoun
   d. Grocott

95. The structures that are stained red in Image 14.25 can also be demonstrated with:

   a. thioflavin T
   b. acridine orange
   c. periodic acid-Schiff
   d. auramine-rhodamine

96. The red structures in Image 14.25 are stained with:

   a. carbol-fuchsin
   b. aldehyde fuchsin
   c. crystal violet
   d. Congo red

97. In order to be demonstrated by the technique illustrated in Image 14.25, the red-stained structures must have:

   a. ionizing ability
   b. acid-fastness
   c. thick cell walls
   d. aldehyde groups

98. A problem will occur in the stain illustrated in Image 14.25 if the:

   a. sections dry after the carbol-fuchsin
   b. carbol-fuchsin is prepared from pararosaniline
   c. acid-alcohol is removed with tap water
   d. a wetting agent is added to the carbol-fuchsin

99. A false-negative stain might occur in the procedure illustrated in Image 14.25 if the tissue were fixed in:

   a. B-5 solution
   b. Bouin solution
   c. Carnoy solution
   d. neutral-buffered formalin

100. The red-stained structures in the illustration in Image 14.25 are most likely:

    a. *Candida albicans*
    b. *Treponema pallidum*
    c. *Mycobacterium tuberculosis*
    d. *Giardia lamblia*

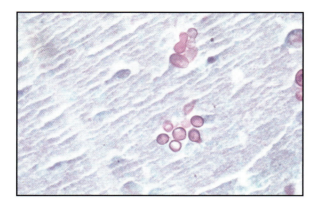

Image 14.26
This image pertains to questions 101–104.

101. Of the following, the artifact seen in Image 14.26 can be caused by:

    a. static electricity
    b. cutting too fast
    c. too little knife tilt
    d. not chilling the block

102. The artifact seen in Image 14.26 might be prevented in the future by:

    a. increasing the flotation bath temperature
    b. increasing the processing times
    c. decreasing the knife tilt
    d. rechilling the block

103. Of the following, the artifact seen in Image 14.26 can be caused by:

    a. a cold flotation bath
    b. overprocessing of the tissue
    c. calcium present in the tissue
    d. aggressive facing of the block

104. The artifact seen in Image 14.26 might be prevented in the future by:

    a. facing the block less aggressively
    b. decalcifying the tissue before processing
    c. increasing the knife tilt
    d. shortening the processing times

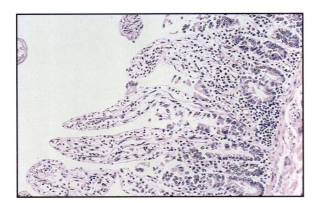

Image 14.27

This image pertains to questions 105–109.

105. The problem seen in Image 14.27 is the result of:

    a. autolysis
    b. poor microtomy
    c. a hot flotation bath
    d. overprocessing

106. The problem demonstrated in Image 14.27 probably could have been prevented if the:

    a. dehydration step had begun with 50% alcohol
    b. specimen had been fixed immediately after removal
    c. temperature of the infiltrating paraffin had been decreased
    d. paraffin sections had been floated on a cooler flotation bath

107. The artifact seen in Image 14.27 is most frequently seen in which of the following specimens?

    a. colonoscopy
    b. post-mortem
    c. surgical removal
    d. endoscopic biopsy

108. The stain used in Image 14.27 is most likely the:

    a. H&E
    b. Giemsa
    c. alcian blue
    d. mucicarmine

109. The tissue component most affected by the problem shown in Image 14.27 is called the:

    a. lamina propria
    b. muscularis externa
    c. epithelium
    d. adventitia

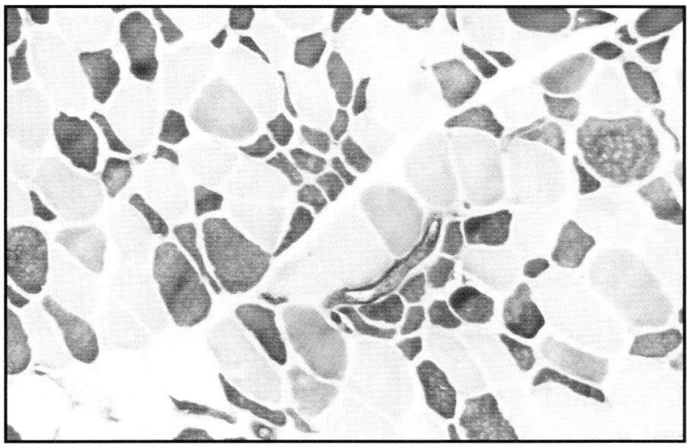

Image 14.28

This image pertains to questions 110–115.

110. The tissue shown in Image 14.28 is:

   a. skeletal muscle
   b. smooth muscle
   c. adrenal gland
   d. thyroid

111. The stain shown in Image 14.28 is most likely the:

   a. NADH diaphorase
   b. acid phosphatase
   c. phosphorylase
   d. ATPase

112. The stain shown in Image 14.28 was done at pH 4.2. The most darkly stained fibers are:

   a. type I
   b. type IIA
   c. type IIB
   d. type IIC

113. The final reaction product in the technique shown in Image 14.28 is:

   a. calcium phosphate
   b. cobalt phosphate
   c. calcium sulfide
   d. cobalt sulfide

114. The technique in Image 14.28 involves:

   a. self-colored substrate
   b. metallic impregnation
   c. metallic substitution
   d. molecular rearrangement

115. The enzyme involved in the technique shown in Image 14.28 below belongs to which of the following classes?

   a. lipases
   b. hydrolases
   c. transferases
   d. oxidoreductases

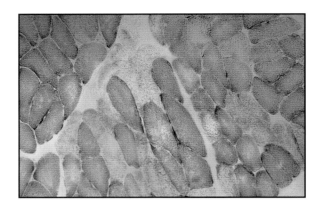

Image 14.29

This image pertains to questions 116–123.

116. The tissue in Image 14.29 is:

    a. skeletal muscle
    b. smooth muscle
    c. adrenal gland
    d. thyroid

117. The stain shown in Image 14.29 is most likely the:

    a. NADH diaphorase
    b. acid phosphatase
    c. phosphorylase
    d. ATPase

118. The enzyme involved in the technique shown in Image 14.29 belongs to which of the following classes?

    a. lipases
    b. hydrolases
    c. transferase
    d. oxidoreductases

119. Which of the following muscle fiber types is stained darker blue in Image 14.29?

    a. I
    b. IIA
    c. IIB
    d. IIC

120. The final reaction product associated with the technique shown in Image 14.29 is:

    a. cobalt sulfide
    b. azo dye
    c. formazan
    d. amylose

121. The reaction shown in Image 14.29 is dependent upon:

    a. metal salt precipitation
    b. insoluble azo dye production
    c. the transfer of hydrogen
    d. the use of substituted naphthols

122. The technique shown in Image 14.29 depends on the use of:

    a. 8-micrometer paraffin sections
    b. frozen sections of unfixed tissue
    c. fixation following frozen sectioning
    d. antigen-retrieval solutions

123. The technique illustrated in Image 14.29 will demonstrate Z-band material, sarcoplasmic reticulum, and:

    a. lysosomes
    b. microtubules
    c. euchromatin
    d. mitochondria

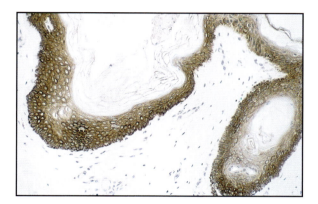

Image 14.30

This image pertains to questions 124–129.

124. The tissue in Image 14.30 is:

    a. tongue
    b. esophagus
    c. cervix
    d. skin

125. The stain in Image 14.30 is most likely a(n):

    a. Fontana-Masson
    b. immunoperoxidase
    c. Grimelius
    d. ATPase

126. The brown-stained tissue structure in Image 14.30 is the:

    a. epithelium
    b. adventitia
    c. muscularis externa
    d. lamina propria

127. The antibody used in the stain shown in Image 14.30 was most likely:

   a. Factor VIII
   b. cytokeratin
   c. vimentin
   d. S-100

128. The chromagen used in Image 14.30 was most likely:

   a. AEC
   b. PAP
   c. DAB
   d. FITC

129. The brown-stained structure in Image 14.30 is known as the:

   a. endothelium
   b. hypodermis
   c. dermis
   d. epidermis

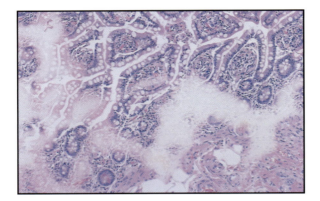

Image 14.31

130. The problem seen in Image 14.31 could be caused by:

   a. poor flotation technique
   b. too much heat during processing
   c. inadequate infiltration with paraffin
   d. incomplete drying of the cut section

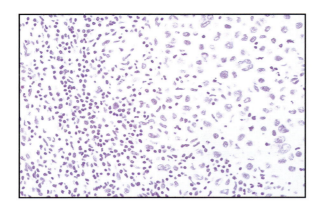

Image 14.32

This image pertains to questions 131–135.

131. The technique in Image 14.32 is most likely the:

    a. Feulgen
    b. Giemsa
    c. methyl green-pyronin
    d. periodic acid-Schiff

132. The tissue component demonstrated by the technique illustrated in Image 14.32 is:

    a. ribonucleic acid
    b. deoxyribonucleic acid
    c. nuclear membrane
    d. nuclear pores

133. The most critical step in the procedure illustrated in Image 14.32 is that of:

    a. reduction
    b. oxidation
    c. hydrolysis
    d. impregnation

134. Which of the following reagents is responsible for the rose color in the technique shown in Image 14.32?

    a. mucicarmine
    b. carbol-fuchsin
    c. Congo red
    d. Schiff

135. Which of the following fixatives will impair the reaction illustrated in Image 14.32?

    a. buffered formalin
    b. Bouin
    c. Zenker
    d. B-5

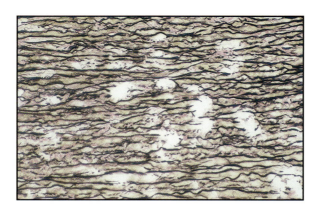

Image 14.33

This image pertains to questions 136–140.

136. The artifact shown in Image 14.33 is most likely the result of:

    a. prolonged formalin fixation
    b. aggressive facing of the block
    c. too hot a flotation bath
    d. air bubbles trapped under the section

137. The artifact shown in Image 14.33 could most likely be prevented in the future by:

    a. decreasing the fixation time
    b. lowering the temperature of the embedding paraffin
    c. facing the paraffin block less aggressively
    d. shortening the time required for processing

138. The artifact shown in Image 14.33 is most likely to occur on tissue that has been subjected to prolonged:

    a. fixation in formalin
    b. wet tissue storage
    c. dehydration
    d. slide drying

139. On which of the following tissues is the artifact shown in Image 14.33 most likely to occur?

    a. lymph node
    b. kidney
    c. uterus
    d. breast

140. The stain shown in the illustration in Image 14.33 is the:

    a. Verhoeff-van Gieson
    b. Gomori aldehyde fuchsin
    c. Grocott methenamine silver
    d. Muller-Mowry colloidal iron

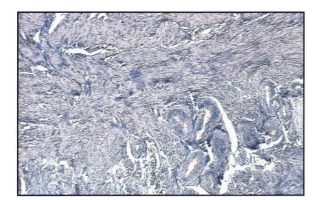

Image 14.34

This image pertains to questions 141–146.

141. The primary problem seen in the Masson trichrome stain in Image 14.34 is the lack of staining in the:

    a. nuclei
    b. collagen
    c. erythrocytes
    d. muscle

142. The problem seen in the Masson trichrome stain in Image 14.34 could most likely be corrected by:

    a. drying the sections longer
    b. increasing the deparaffinizing time
    c. changing to new staining solutions
    d. acidifying the mounting medium

143. The problem seen in the Masson trichrome stain shown in Image 14.34 was most likely the result of:

    a. improper drying of the sections
    b. incomplete deparaffinization
    c. pathologically altered collagen
    d. old or depleted reagents

144. In the stain illustrated in Image 14.34, the absence of some red stained tissue elements indicate:

    a. excellent staining quality
    b. a depleted staining solution
    c. an underdifferentiated stain
    d. the absence of blood vessels

145. The tissue shown in Image 14.34 has been stained with the Masson trichrome. After reviewing this slide, the technician should:

    a. repeat the stain using heat
    b. label the slide and sign it out
    c. decolorize and restain the section
    d. repeat the stain, ensuring mordanting in Bouin

146. The smooth muscle in Image 14.34 most likely should be stained:

    a. red
    b. green
    c. yellow
    d. blue

Image-Based Questions Answer Key

The following items have been identified as appropriate for both entry-level histologic technicians and histotechnologists.

1. c	38. c	75. a	112. a
2. c	39. c	76. c	113. d
3. b	40. b	77. c	114. c
4. b	41. c	78. a	115. b
5. c	42. c	79. b	116. a
6. c	43. a	80. d	117. a
7. c	44. d	81. c	118. d
8. a	45. b	82. a	119. a
9. b	46. d	83. b	120. c
10. d	47. b	84. c	121. c
11. c	48. d	85. c	122. b
12. d	49. b	86. d	123. d
13. d	50. c	87. a	124. d
14. b	51. c	88. b	125. b
15. a	52. a	89. c	126. a
16. a	53. a	90. b	127. b
17. c	54. b	91. d	128. c
18. c	55. d	92. d	129. d
19. b	56. c	93. a	130. d
20. a	57. a	94. c	131. a
21. c	58. b	95. d	132. b
22. b	59. c	96. a	133. c
23. d	60. a	97. b	134. d
24. d	61. b	98. a	135. b
25. a	62. d	99. c	136. b
26. a	63. c	100. c	137. c
27. c	64. b	101. b	138. c
28. c	65. b	102. c	139. a
29. d	66. c	103. b	140. a
30. b	67. a	104. d	141. d
31. c	68. d	105. a	142. c
32. d	69. b	106. b	143. d
33. b	70. c	107. b	144. b
34. b	71. a	108. a	145. d
35. c	72. b	109. c	146. a
36. b	73. c	110. a	
37. a	74. d	111. d	